Making the Right Decision:
A TRIAGE CURRICULUM

2nd Edition

ISBN# 0-935890-66-1

Table of Contents

SECTION 1: BASIC TRIAGE CONCEPTS
Chapter 1: Triage Overview 3
Chapter 2: Triage Assessment 17
Chapter 3: Triage Documentation 39
Chapter 4: Legal Issues 47
Chapter 5: Customer Service 59
Chapter 6: Cultural & Religious Considerations 69
Chapter 7: Violence 79
Chapter 8: Disaster Triage 89

SECTION 2: CLINICAL CONCEPTS 99
Chapter 9: Universal Triage Parameters 103
Chapter 10: Abdomen/Pelvis 113
Chapter 11: Abuse and Neglect 127
Chapter 12: Back 141
Chapter 13: Bites and Stings 149
Chapter 14: Burns 157
Chapter 15: Chest 163
Chapter 16: Cold-Related Conditions 171
Chapter 17: Confusion 177
Chapter 18: Ear 183
Chapter 19: Extremity 189
Chapter 20: Eye 199
Chapter 21: Fever 209
Chapter 22: Head 215
Chapter 23: Heat-related Conditions 229
Chapter 24: Mouth 235
Chapter 25: Neck 241
Chapter 26: Nose 249
Chapter 27: Obstetrical Complaints 255
Chapter 28: Psychiatric Complaints 263
Chapter 29: Respiratory 273
Chapter 30: Seizure 285
Chapter 31: Sexual Assault 293

Chapter 32: Skin Problems 299

Chapter 33: Surface Wounds 305

Chapter 34: Throat 313

Chapter 35: Toxicities 319

Chapter 36: Trauma 327

Chapter 37: Advanced Triage Exercises 341

SECTION 3
Glossary 351

SECTION 4: APPENDICES
Appendix A: Triage Assessment Competency Guidelines 355

Appendix B: Adult Learning 357

Appendix C: CECH Application 363

Appendix D: Comprehensive Triage Standards 367

Appendix E: Sample Documentation Forms 373

Acknowledgments

The Emergency Nurses Association (ENA) would like to extend its appreciation to the following people for the development of *Making the Right Decision: A Triage Curriculum, 2nd edition.*

Editor

Lorene Newberry, RN, MS, CEN
Clinical Nurse Specialist, Emergency Services
WellStar Health Systems
Marietta, GA

Reviewers

Lisa R. Ray, RN
Emergency Nursing Consultant
Atlanta, GA

Kevin Daniel, RN
Clinician, Emergency Department
Northside Hospital
Atlanta, GA

Anita Efremov, RN, BSN
Manager Emergency Services and Central Clinical
  Admissions
Wellstar Cobb Hospital
Austell, GA

Contributing Authors

David Eitel, MD, MBA
Department of Emergency Medicine
The York Hospital, WellSpan Health
York, PA

Nicki Gilboy, RN, MS, CEN
Nurse Educator, Emergency Department
Brigham and Women's Hospital
Boston, MA

Paula Tanabe, RN, PhD, CEN, CCRN
Advanced Practice Nurse, Emergency Department
Northwestern Memorial Hospital
Chicago, IL

Debbie Travers, RN, MSN, CEN
Triage Nurse, Emergency Department
University of North Carolina Hospitals
Chapel Hill, NC

Staff Liaisons

Jennifer Heidenreich
Senior Graphic Designer
ENA

Carla M. Rea, MBA
Member Services Manager
ENA

George Velianoff, DNS RN, CHE
Chief Operating Officer
ENA

MAKING THE RIGHT DECISION: A TRIAGE CURRICULUM
FIRST EDITION

SECTION EDITORS

Daniel R. Bleyhl, RN, BSN, CEN
DB Consulting
Omaha, NE

Karen Lorbert Chung, RN, MSN, CEN
Advanced Clinical Educator, Nursing Education, Staff
  Development and Training
Children's National Medical Center
Washington, DC

Zeb Koran, RN, MSN, CEN, CCRN
Director: Educational Services
ENA

Sonia K. Liberatore, RN, MS
Nurse Manager and QA Coordinator, Radiology
Strong Memorial Hospital Rochester, NY

Emily Magid, RN, MSN, CEN
Emergency Clinical Nurse Specialist
San Jose Medical Center
San Jose, CA

Nurse Editor

Susan Moore, RN, MS, CEN, CCRN
Staff Nurse, Emergency Department
Washoe Medical Center
Reno, NV

Contributing Authors

Judith M. Belle-Isle, RN, BSN
Nuclear Cardiology
University of Rochester Medical Center
Rochester, NY

Daniel R. Bleyhl, RN, BSN, CEN
DB Consulting
Omaha, NE

Catherine A. Carrico, RN, BSN, CEN
Staff Nurse
Nebraska Methodist/Children's Hospital
Omaha, NE

Karen Lorbert Chung, RN, MSN, CEN
Advanced Clinical Educator, Nursing Education, Staff
  Development and Training
Children's National Medical Center Washington, DC

Bonnie A. Coons, RN, BSN, CEN
Nurse Leader/Management
University of Rochester Medical Center
Rochester, NY

Carol Crane, RN, MSN, MBA
Psychiatric Consultation Liaison, Nursing
Strong Memorial Hospital
Rochester, NY

Ann Donze, RN, MS(N)
Neonatal Nurse Practitioner
St. Louis Children's Hospital
St. Louis, MO

Martha R. Dorn, MD
Chief of Emergency Services
Palo Alto Vetuana Medical Center
Stanford University
Palo Alto, CA

Charose James, RN, BSN, CEN
Staff Nurse
Nebraska Methodist Hospital
Omaha, NE

Zeb Koran, RN, MSN, CEN, CCRN
Director: Educational Services
ENA

Laura L. Kuensting, RN, MSN(R)
Educational Specialist, Emergency Services
Cardinal Glennon Children's Hospital St. Louis, MO

Judith M. Landvatter, RN, BSN, EMT-P
Outreach Education Coordinator, Emergency Services
St. Louis Children's Hospital St. Louis, MO

Sonia K. Liberatore, RN, MS
Nurse Manager and QA Coordinator, Radiology
Strong Memorial Hospital
Rochester, NY

Emily Magid, RN, MSN, CEN
Emergency Clinical Nurse Specialist
San Jose Medical Center
San Jose, CA

Sandra Manjasek, JD
Attorney-at-Law
Gosney, Manjasek, and Moore

Geralynn M. Sanders, RN, BSN
Staff Nurse, Emergency Services
Cardinal Clennon Children's Hospital
St. Louis, MO
Alice M. Washburn, RN
Staff Nurse/Case Manager, Emergency Department
Nebraska Methodist Hospital Omaha, NE

Karla J. Ziesemer, RN, CEN
Staff Nurse, Emergency Department
Nebraska Methodist Hospital
Omaha, NE

Learning Assessment Authors

Sue Barnason, RN, PhD, CEN, CCRN
Clinical Nurse Specialist, Emergency
Department & Critical Care Bryan Memorial Hospital
Lincoln, NE

Robert W. Ready, RN, MN, CEN
Clinical Manager, Children's Emergency Department
Rhode Island Hospital
Providence, RI

Preface

Triage: Making the Right Decision was developed as an educational program to train nurses in the art and science of triage. The program stresses the importance of working with an experienced triage nurse and functioning within guidelines established by state practice acts and facility constraints for the learner's practice location. The first edition has been revised to assure clinical relevance and content accuracy. Several changes have been made to enhance usability and facilitate the learning process.

- Three manuals from the first edition have been consolidated into two resource manuals—one for the preceptor and one for the learner.
  -Content from the learner manual is replicated verbatim in the preceptor manual.
  -Learning assessment questions and clinical application questions for each chapter are found in the Learner Resource Manual.
    ∎ These questions are replicated with answer keys for learning assessment questions in the preceptor manual.
  -Clinical application exercises provided for each chapter challenge the learner to apply content from the chapter to their specific practice and the facility where they work. Answers are facility specific.
- The preceptor manual contains a glossary of terms, ENA practice standards for the competent triage nurse, CECH forms, information on adult learning, and sample triage forms

Each resource manual contains eight chapters that address basic triage concepts, 28 clinical chapters, and one chapter of advanced triage exercises. The format for each manual uses large outside margins that provide instructions for the preceptor. Margins are blank in the learner manual for notes.

- New chapters address the patient with obstetrical complaints, respiratory problems, and the victim of sexual assault.
- The previous chapter on mouth and throat has been split into two separate chapters.
- Focus for the chest chapter has been changed to the patient with chest pain and other cardiac-type problems. (Respiratory problems are addressed in a separate chapter.)
- The old chapter on skin and soft tissue has been split into separate chapters on bites and stings, burns, skin problems, and surface wounds.
- Chapters on abuse and neglect as well as trauma have been moved to Clinical Chapters.
  -Trauma to the head, neck, chest, abdomen are discussed in the Trauma Chapter. Isolated orthopedic injuries are discussed in the Extremity Chapter.
- A 5-level triage system has been incorporated in several chapters.

Triage is one of the more challenging, albeit less glamorous, roles the emergency nurse has. This 'subspecialty' of emergency nursing affects patient care and patient flow through the entire emergency department. Triage is an area that is high-volume, high-risk, and problem-prone. Successful triage requires the nurse to have a sound knowledge base, excellent clinical skills, and superb customer service skills. This book is designed for registered nurses with a minimum of six months experience in emergency nursing. The learner should work with an experienced triage nurse to maximize learning. Content is intended as a framework for education and orientation to triage. However, triage decisions are individual and often complex. Consequently, information in these texts must be adapted to meet individual facilities and state practice acts.

To the triage nurse . . . emergency nursing's unsung hero.

BASIC TRIAGE CONCEPTS

This section provides a basic foundation on which to build your skill as a triage nurse. Triage is much more than taking vital signs and asking the patient what is wrong. Many other skills are required of the triage nurse. Understanding these areas will enable you to function competently and effectively in various roles that are all part of triage. Specific areas covered are:

- Overview of triage
- Assessment
- Documentation
- Legal issues
- Customer service
- Cultural and religious considerations
- Violence
- Disaster triage

Ability to function effectively in the triage role requires a basic foundation of knowledge, skill, and flexibility. As you study each chapter in this section, ask yourself how it applies to your current work situation. Work with your preceptor to mold these concepts to your needs and to the department in which you work. Use the information to build a knowledge base that makes the move to more complex clinical concepts a smooth journey.

Triage Overview *chapter 1*

OBJECTIVES

After completing this chapter, you will be able to:

1. Define triage.

2. Describe three primary objectives of an emergency department (ED) triage system.

3. Define three acuity categories.

4. Describe four roles of the triage nurse.

RESOURCES

- Patient flow diagram showing the process from arrival to disposition

- Institutional statistics for emergent, urgent, and nonurgent patient visits

- Triage-related policies: Triage, mission statements, triage acuity categories, waiting room reassessment, infection control, telephone advice, nurse calls, workers' compensation insurance, nonemergency screening procedures

- Triage protocols

- Maps and telephone lists

- Patient teaching resources

- Performance improvement monitoring tools, reporting mechanisms, and policies related to these activities at triage

INTRODUCTION

The process of triage, recognized as a foundation of emergency nursing, is an integral process in the ED. Triage requires both simple and complex knowledge. The process may be simple and straightforward for some patients but complicated and even controversial for others. This chapter provides an overview of triage concepts, definitions, and roles to establish a common language to be used as you progress through this program.

The term "triage" is derived from the French verb "trier" that refers to sorting or choosing. Simply put, triage is the process of sorting or classifying patients according to urgency of condition or compliant. Effective triage gets the patient to the right place at the right time with the right care provider. Triage is the first decision point in care of the emergency patient. The patient presents to the ED where information is elicited to determine the nature of the problem as well as the urgency with which the problem should be evaluated and treated. A priority of care is assigned to the patient, and the patient is then sent to the appropriate area or provider for further evaluation and treatment. Incorrect identification of the patient's problem can delay treatment and may adversely affect outcome. For example, a patient who complains of jaw pain may be incorrectly sent to the dental clinic if the nurse does not consider other causes of this pain, such as myocardial infarction.

During World War I, triage was used to separate soldiers with the most salvageable injuries from those who required more extensive care. This process allowed rapid treatment for those who could be treated and quickly returned to the battlefield. Triage enabled military personnel to focus resources on soldiers who were most likely to survive and could return to battle. Triage appeared in civilian hospitals during the late 1950s and early 1960s in response to increasing volume of patients and use of the ED for treatment of nonurgent conditions (Rund & Rausch, 1981). In the civilian arena, triage was used to identify patients with an immediate threat to life or limb. As the population increases and number of ED visits continues to climb, problems with overcrowding only highlight the need for an effective triage system.

Today, triage can be divided into two basic categories: Nondisaster and multicasualty (or disaster). Both types include classification and acuity systems for treatment and transport; however, the purpose of each type is very different.

- *Nondisaster triage* is used to provide the best care for each patient.

- *Multicasualty/disaster triage* is designed to provide the most effective care for the greatest number of patients. Disaster triage, or military triage, is primarily oriented for use in the prehospital arena. Delayed transport is used to prevent overloading the ED and to maximize use of available resources.

EMERGENCY DEPARTMENT TRIAGE SYSTEMS

Triage systems are as varied as the EDs that use them. These systems are designed to meet the needs of the user and to function effectively in rapidly changing health care institutions. Triage systems may differ in staffing, documentation, triage categories, assessment parameters, reassessment guidelines, and treatment protocols. Despite these variations, triage systems generally fall into three common types identified by Thompson and Dains (1982) (see Table 1-1).

Table 1-1. ED Triage Systems			
Type and Name	**Staffing**	**Urgency Categories**	**Protocols and Treatment**
I: Traffic Director	Nonprofessional	Two: Emergent or urgent	None
II: Spot-Check	RN or MD	Three: Emergent, urgent, delayed	Variable
III: Comprehensive	RN	Four	Driven by protocols

Type I: Traffic Director or Non-Nurse Triage

Non-nurse triage is the most basic system used. Nonlicensed personnel, such as a secretary, department clerk, registration clerk, technician, or nursing aide, obtain minimal information—usually the patient's name and chief complaint. An impression of how sick the patient looks is used with this information to determine if the patient has an emergent or urgent condition. There are no established standards or protocols for care, and documentation is very limited.

Inherent problems with this system relate to superficial assessment of potentially serious problems as well as violation of applicable regulatory mandates. The Emergency Treatment and Active Labor Act (EMTALA) requires an initial medical screening examination (MSE) for patients who seek treatment in the ED. The MSE is used to rule out an emergent medical condition *before* asking the patient any financial information. With nonlicensed personnel making first contact, there is greater risk that the patient may be asked financial questions before completion of the MSE. (Refer to Chapter 4: Legal Issues for more discussion of EMTALA.) Secondly, this system does not meet standards established by the Emergency Nurses Association (ENA) for comprehensive triage (Appendix A).

Type II: Spot-Check Triage

A "quick look" by a registered nurse (RN) or physician is the basis of this system. This system is also called advanced triage because licensed professional personnel perform this rapid assessment. Limited subjective, objective, and historical information is obtained prior to making a determination of acuity. The goal of this system is to ensure that patients with the most serious illness or injury are treated first. Three primary triage categories are used: emergent, urgent, and nonurgent. Protocol use varies from institution to institution. Formal assessment criteria and documentation requirements also vary by facility.

Type III: Comprehensive Triage

This system encompasses all aspects of the triage process. It is the most advanced of the common ED triage systems and is supported by ENA's Practice Standard for Triage (Appendix B). Registered nurses with appropriate education and experience assess and prioritize patients using various data and predetermined guidelines. Subjective and objective data considered in concert with past medical history, health status, psychosocial components, and health behaviors are used to identify physiological, educational, and primary health needs (Thompson & Dains, 1982). Four or five categories may be used for patient prioritization.

One advantage of this system is consistency. Using protocols and written standards for assessment and documentation minimizes variability between users. Written standards for assessment, planning, and intervention are used to guide the triage process. Protocols are used to initiate diagnostic tests, select treatments, and re-evaluate the patient.

Other Triage Systems

Unique characteristics of an individual ED, facility, or location have led to variations in triage systems. Many facilities combine two of the three basic ED triage systems. For example, a two-tiered triage system may utilize the Spot-Check System as the first step with the Comprehensive System as the second tier. This system has advantages for some high-volume EDs. The triage nurse greets the patient on arrival, determines chief complaint, and performs a primary survey to determine whether the patient can wait for further assessment. Patients with an emergent condition or emergent complaint are taken immediately to a treatment area. The second triage nurse completes the triage assessment for patients who can wait. The first triage nurse may be called the screening nurse or initial triage nurse, whereas the second nurse is referred to as the assessment nurse. Some EDs use licensed practical nurses or paramedics to perform initial triage; however, ENA does not support this.

Other triage systems use separate staff to triage ambulatory patients and those brought by ambulance. An external triage nurse is responsible for assessment of ambulatory patients while an internal nurse evaluates ambulance patients, and assigns a bed or treatment area.

TRIAGE CONCEPTS

Various labels may be used to identify the triage nurse including triage officer, triage agent, and triageur; however, the preferred term is triage nurse. Just as ENA recommends a specially educated RN (ENA, 1999) perform triage; use of the term triage nurse is also encouraged. Therefore, throughout this text, the term triage nurse identifies the RN who performs triage. Aspects of triage such as vital signs, visual acuity examination, and patient transport may be delegated to other appropriately trained staff; however, the triage nurse is still responsible for the patient. State practice acts and institutional policies determine what tasks can be delegated and to whom they can be delegated. Critical thinking skills enable the triage nurse to assimilate data from various sources and set priorities for patient care based on particular circumstances of the patient and ED at that time.

Triage requires the nurse to have clinical knowledge as well as the ability to manage multiple tasks. The triage nurse affects not only those patients in the waiting area, but also patient flow through the entire department. These complex and diverse requirements make triage daunting to those without experience. Specific objectives of the triage system are highlighted in Table 1-2. Time-tested principles that assist the triage nurse in accomplishing these objectives include the following:

- Greet patients and identify yourself as the triage nurse.

- Maintain patient confidentiality in all interactions.

- Maintain visual access of incoming patients even while interviewing others.

- Ensure flow of information between triage personnel and patients in the waiting area as well as between the triage and treatment areas.

- Know the institution's triage system and your own limitations. Remember the primary objectives of the triage role.

- Use available resources to maintain the appropriate standard of care.

Table 1-2. Primary Objectives for ED Triage Systems

- Identify patients who require immediate care.
- Determine the appropriate area for treatment.
- Facilitate patient flow through the ED and avoid unnecessary congestion.
- Provide continued assessment and reassessment of arriving and waiting patients.
- Provide information and referrals to patients and families.
- Allay patient and family anxiety.
- Enhance public relations.

(ENA, 1992)

Acuity Categories

Patients are assessed by the triage nurse then sorted by patient acuity. Acuity refers to severity of illness or injury as well as the potential for complications related to the illness or injury. Complications include adverse physical outcomes and undue suffering. The primary goal of triage is to identify patients who require immediate treatment for life-threatening conditions. The triage nurse's second goal is to sort or prioritize patients according to identified acuity. Determination of acuity is made using a system of two to five acuity levels. A number, letter, or name may identify a specific level. Specific criteria for each level include the degree to which the complaint is life-threatening, risk for short-term complications, time parameters for requisite treatment, amount of patient or family suffering, and availability of treatment areas and providers.

> **Key Concept**
> The primary goal of triage is to identify life-threatening conditions. The second goal is to prioritize patients according to acuity.

There are many rating systems used for triage acuity. In the annual ENA survey of EDs in 1996, managers reported the type of triage acuity scales used in their departments. 64% used a 3-level scale, 6% used a 4-level scale, 10% used a 5-level scale, and 20% didn't respond to the question or had no triage rating system (ENA, 1996).

For simplicity, 3-level and 5-level triage scales are presented here. In 3-level triage, the primary acuity categories are emergent, urgent and nonurgent.

- Emergent: Involves an immediate threat to life, vision, or limb
- Urgent: Requires prompt care, but will not cause loss of life, vision, or limb if untreated for several hours
- Nonurgent: Requires evaluation and treatment, but time is not a critical factor

Table 1-3 provides an overview of these categories. Several time-critical situations and general examples are included; however, these examples should not be considered all-inclusive or the standard for each level. It is also important to remember that a change in the patient's condition may require change in the acuity level.

Table 1-3. Triage Acuity System Using Three Levels		
Acuity	**Reassessment**	**Examples**
Emergent	Continuous	Cardiopulmonary arrest, severe respiratory distress, major burns, major or multisystem trauma, massive hemorrhage, coma, crushing substernal chest pain, anaphylaxis, high-risk needle stick requiring postexposure prophylaxis
Urgent	Every 30 to 60 minutes	Abdominal pain, multiple fractures, asthma, open fracture, renal calculi
Nonurgent	Every 1 to 2 hours	Rash, cystitis, sprains, minor lacerations, chronic headache, vaginal discharge, sexually transmitted disease

Five-level triage scales are widely used in Australia, Canada and the United Kingdom (Australasian College for Emergency Medicine, 1997; Beveridge, Ducharme, Janes, Beaulieu, & Walter, 1999; Manchester Triage Group, 1997). Research in Australia and Canada indicate that the scales have excellent reliability (consistent assignment of triage categories across nurses) and validity (strong association of triage levels with outcomes and resource use) (Jelinek & Little, 1996; Beveridge, Ducharme, Janes, Beaulieu, & Walter, 1999). The Australian National Triage Scale (NTS) utilizes colors to exemplify the urgency of the patient's condition: resuscitation (red), emergency (orange), urgent (green), semi-urgent (blue) and non-urgent (white). Triage nurses assign acuity ratings based on the time frame in which a provider should see the patients. For example, a resuscitation patient should be seen immediately, and a semi-urgent patient within one hour.

The Canadian Triage and Acuity Scale (CTAS), although independently derived, is based on time objectives similar to the NTS, and includes the following categories: level 1 (resuscitation), level 2 (emergent), level 3 (urgent), level 4 (less urgent) and level 5 (non urgent). The National Emergency Nurses Affiliation (NENA) and the Canadian Association of Emergency Physicians (CAEP) have endorsed the CTAS as the standard for ED triage. Canadian hospitals must use the CTAS data element for mandatory reporting of all ED visits to the Canadian government (CAEP, 2001).

The Manchester Triage Scale, from Great Britian, is also five levels, with categories as follows: level 1 (immediate- red), level 2 (very urgent- orange) level 3 (urgent-yellow) level 4 (standard- green), and level 5 (non-urgent-blue). The system is organized by chief complaint. The triage nurse selects the appropriate presentational flow-diagram (complaint algorithm) and proceeds to take the patient through a series of predetermined questions that are specific to that complaint. For example, a level 2 chest pain patient is one with severe chest heaviness, and a level 4 chest pain patient is one with mild chest pain for several days

A new 5-level triage acuity and resource scale called the Emergency Severity Index (ESI), has been developed in the United States. The ESI stratifies patients into five explicitly defined, mutually exclusive categories: from level 1 (dying patient) to level 5 (simple problem, stable patient). Two emergency physicians, Richard Wuerz and David Eitel, are responsible for the conceptual breakthrough and the flowchart-based triage algorithm that exists today (Gilboy, Travers & Wuerz, 1999). Unlike other triage systems ESI categorizes emergency patients by both acuity and expected resource needs. Acuity is defined in terms of the stability of the patient's vital functions (for example, the ABC's of airway, breathing and circulation). Expected resource needs refer to the number of resources a patient will likely consume before a disposition is reached. Research conducted at a variety of Emergency Departments in the U.S. has demonstrated that the Emergency Severity Index is both reliable and valid (Wuerz, Milne, Eitel, Traver & Gilboy, 2000; Wuerz, Travers, Gilboy, Eitel, Rosenau, Yazhari, 2001). The strong inter-rater reliability of this tool allows institutions to compare their own case mix with other institutions as well as track changes over time in their own ED. Operating performance indicators and a variety of outcomes by triage class can then be tracked and analyzed within, and across, Emergency Departments using the ESI, since the assignments are reliable.

In using the ESI, triage nurses first make judgments about a triage class (level 1 or 2) based on the urgency of the patient's condition, and then decide on a triage class (level 3, 4 or 5) based upon the likely number of resources necessary to get the patient through the ED to a disposition. Vital signs are used as a consideration to potentially up-triage patients to a higher triage class. The ESI algorithm uses four decision points to determine triage category, as shown in Figure x. Each box asks a specific question. Starting at the top of the algorithm, the first box asks "is the patient dying"? If the answer is yes then the patient is categorized as an ESI level 1. If the answer is no, then the next decision is made – "is this a patient who shouldn't wait more than a few minutes to be seen"? For example, the patient who presents to triage with active chest pain would fall into this category and would therefore be rated as a level 2. If, on the other hand, the patient can wait, then the next decision must be made – predicting the number of institutional resources that this patient will need or consume in order to reach a disposition. A patient who requires no additional resources is classified as a level 5. An example of this level is a request for a prescription refill. A level 4 patient presumably requires one resource, and a level 3

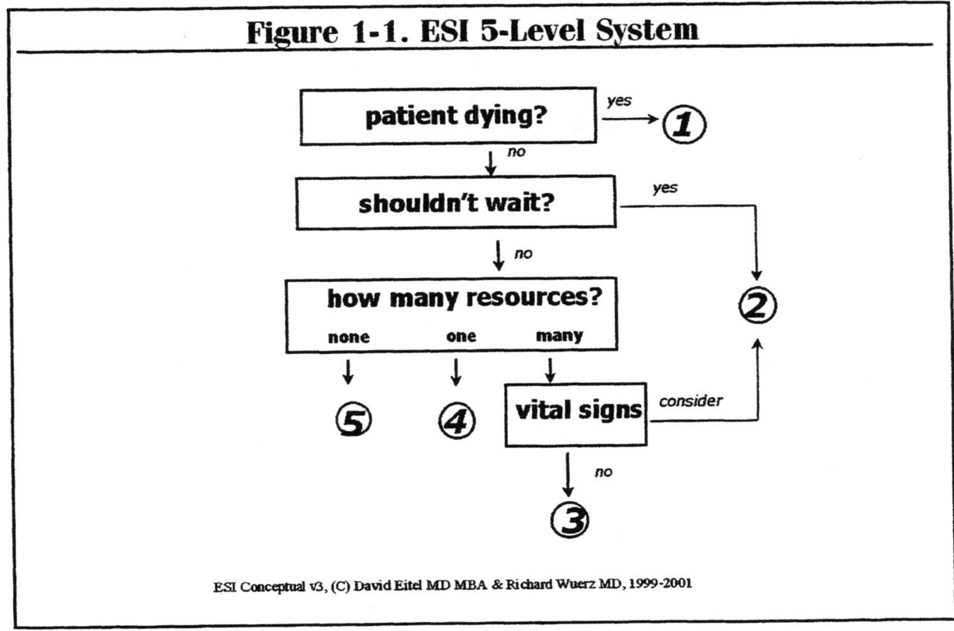

Figure 1-1. ESI 5-Level System

ESI Conceptual v3, (C) David Eitel MD MBA & Richard Wuerz MD, 1999-2001

patient is expected to require two or more resources. If a patient requires two or more resources the triage nurse must next determine if the patient's vital signs are a concern. If the vital signs fall outside a set of predetermined parameters, then the nurse has the option to up-triage the patient to a level 2.

Additional examples of level 2 patients are provided here.

- Shortness of breath, increasing over 2 days, mild to moderate respiratory distress, in a patient with a history of colon cancer and oxygen saturation of 91%

- Combative, hostile, homicidal patient accompanied by three police officers

- Right lower quadrant abdominal pain associated with loss of appetite, nausea and vomiting in a patient with no significant past medical history, heart rate of 110 and low grade fever

> **Key Concept**
> **Acuity level may change at any time.**

Mistriage

Mistriage refers to assignment of an acuity level that is higher or lower than necessary for a specific patient. *Over-triage* (or assignment of a higher acuity level than necessary) taxes resources that could be used for patients with more serious illness or injury. Length of stay may also be prolonged by over-triage. *Under-triage* is potentially more serious, because the patient receives an acuity level that is lower than appropriate. Delayed treatment because of under-triage can lead to increased morbidity or mortality. The triage nurse can consult a more experienced triage nurse or physician to facilitate identification of the appropriate acuity level; however, this may delay care.

> **Key Concept**
> **When in doubt about acuity level, choose the higher acuity level to avoid under-triage.**

Protocols

Protocols are used to assign categories, direct diagnostic orders, and initiate therapeutic interventions. Referrals to specific treatment areas and/or providers may also be determined by protocols. Use of protocols minimizes variability by providing consistency from one provider to another. Protocols used in triage include, but are not limited to, administration of antipyretics in febrile patients, ordering x-rays for sprains and fractures, and ordering a urinalysis for patients with primary urinary symptoms or abdominal pain.

TRIAGE RESPONSIBILITIES

Responsibilities assigned to the triage nurse vary from institution to institution. One ED may require the triage nurse to make follow-up calls to emergency patients seen the previous day, while another ED may expect the triage nurse to do chart audits. Geraci (1994) identified 29 physical activities and 26 telephone activities performed by triage nurses in a comprehensive triage setting. Despite these numerous tasks, the triage nurse must always focus on the primary activity or role. In general, most triage nurses are faced with clinical and nonclinical duties. These duties may be clearly identified in a formal job description or they may only be understood as part of the job that is expected by management, colleagues, and patients. Clinical duties include performing the actual triage process, administering medication, assisting patients from cars, and, on rare occasions, performing cardiopulmonary resuscitation. Nonclinical duties vary among facilities, but the most common nonclinical duties are discussed below.

Public Relations

The ED is considered the window to the hospital. For most facilities, it is the only entrance after hours. The triage nurse is often the first health care professional that patients encounter. For the patient, at that moment, the triage nurse represents the ED, the hospital, and often the health care system. A negative experience with the triage nurse can affect how the patient and his or her family view the rest of the visit. The triage nurse must juggle multiple tasks while welcoming new arrivals in a professional, friendly manner. This can be particularly challenging during times of high acuity or high census; however, in today's competitive health care environment, this is an essential function of the triage nurse.

Traffic Director

Not every person who presents to the triage desk is seeking treatment in the ED. Individuals may need directions to other areas of the hospital or want information about a current patient. The triage nurse must manage these situations while maintaining contact with new arrivals. Viewing the position of triage nurse as the gatekeeper for the ED illustrates the impact that triage has on overall flow through the department. Posting effective, universal signs and maps can make this aspect of the triage nurse's role easier.

Nonemergency Screener

Diversification of services offered by the ED has increased the requirement for nonemergency screening. Patients may be screened for referral to occupational health clinics or other treatment areas. Examples of nonemergent activities include drug and alcohol screening for employers and law enforcement officers, blood pressure checks, and follow-up care for minor injuries. Workers' compensation insurance forms and procedures may also be required. For these nonemergency screening requirements, the triage nurse must remember that all patients who present to the ED must receive an MSE as required by EMTALA and facility bylaws–before they are referred away from the ED.

Teacher

Patient teaching may begin at triage and can include basic health concepts, illness and injury prevention, use of the emergency care system, and self-care skills such as first aid for extremity injuries. The triage nurse first determines how receptive the patient and/or family is and then provides appropriate education in a positive, constructive manner. Lectures or judgmental statements should be avoided.

Infection Control

Screening patients at triage for potentially infectious diseases and providing appropriate isolation measures hinders disease transmission. The triage nurse uses basic techniques to prevent the spread of infection, including handwashing, use of personal protective equipment when indicated, and terminal cleaning of the triage area as appropriate.

Telephone

Telephone activities can tax even the most experienced triage nurse when patient census is high or the number of telephone calls is excessive. The triage nurse may be required to receive telephone calls from patients, physicians, and the public as well as to make telephone calls to these same people. Requirements include taking physician orders, notifying physicians or families of patient arrival, and answering questions from patients previously seen in the ED. Managed care organizations may call with authorization information for visits, and pharmacists may call because they cannot read the physician's handwriting on prescriptions. Despite these problems, the goal of the triage nurse is always to determine patient acuity. Using voice mail and dedicated physician lines or rolling the telephone over to another area can help control some of the telephone traffic for the triage nurse.

Crowd Control

Arrival of patients and families in great numbers may require the triage nurse to implement crowd control measures. The triage nurse should maintain a calm, professional demeanor while directing families to registration or asking individuals to move to another location. Situations can quickly escalate in the presence of alcohol, drugs, or uncontrolled anger. It is imperative that the triage nurse know the layout of the triage area and how to quickly summon help. Panic buttons, security personnel in the ED, and a separate area for grieving families can decrease anxiety related to this issue.

Team Member

The triage nurse does not work in a vacuum. As a team member, the triage nurse is responsible for making and communicating triage decisions and interventions. Consultation with colleagues when appropriate is also part of triage. Essential skills for triage nurses are also essential skills for teamwork: communication and leadership. Providing feedback about the triage process to appropriate personnel and groups is another aspect of teamwork required of the triage nurse.

SUMMARY

Triage is simple and complex. Beyond clinical knowledge, understanding the goals of triage, requisite functions, and key concepts helps the triage nurse appropriately assess and treat patients in the triage area.

References

Australasian College for Emergency Medicine. (1994). National triage scale. <u>Emergency Medicine (Australia), 6</u>, 145-146.

Australasian College for Emergency Medicine. (1997). <u>The National Triage Scale: A User Manual</u>. Australia: Author.

Beveridge, R., Ducharme, J., Janes, L., Beaulieu, S., & Walter, S. (1999). Reliability of the Canadian emergency department triage and acuity scale: Interrater agreement. <u>Annals of Emergency Medicine, 34</u>, 155-9.

Canadian Association of Emergency Physicians. <u>http://www.caep.ca/</u>. Accessed May 27, 2001.

Emergency Nurses Association. (1998). <u>Standards of emergency nursing</u> (4th ed.). Park Ridge, IL: Author.

Emergency Nurses Association. (1999). <u>National Emergency Department Database Survey, 1997 Annual Survey</u> Report Summary. Park Ridge, IL: Author.

Geraci, E.B., & Geraci, T.A. (1994). An observational study of the emergency triage nursing role in a managed care facility. <u>Journal of Emergency Nursing, 20</u>(3), 189-194.

Gilboy N, Travers DA, Wuerz RC. (1999). Re-evaluating triage in the new millennium: A comprehensive look at the need for standardization and quality. <u>Journal of Emergency Nursing, 25</u>(6), 468-73.

Jelinek, G.A., Little, M. (1996). Inter-rater reliability of the National Triage Scale over 11,500 simulated occaasions of triage. <u>Emergency Medicine, 8</u>, 226-230.

Jordan, K. (Ed.). (2000). <u>Emergency nursing core curriculum</u> (5th ed.). Philadelphia: Saunders.

Manchester Triage Group. (1997). <u>Emergency Triage</u>. Plymouth: BMJ Publishing Group.

Rund, D., & Rausch, T. (1981). <u>Triage</u>. St.Louis: Mosby-Year Book.

Thompson, J., & Dains, J. (1982). <u>Comprehensive triage</u>. Reston, VA: Reston Publishing.

Wuerz RC, Travers D, Gilboy N, Eitel DR, Rosenau A, Yazhari R. Implementation and refinement of the Emergency Severity Index. <u>Academic Emergency Medicine</u>. 2001; 8(2):170-6.

Wuerz RC, Milne LW, Eitel DR, Travers D, Gilboy N. (2000). Reliability and validity of a new five-level triage instrument. <u>Academic Emergency Medicine, 7</u>(3), 236-242.

1. Identify the triage system category (ND=Nondisaster   MC/D=Multicasualty/disaster) that best describes the following:
   Provides the best care for each individual patient
   Provides the most effective care for the greatest number of patients
   Oriented to the prehospital arena
   Triage decisions are made by a team
   Triage decisions are made by a single triage nurse

2. Which of the following reflects undertriage?
   a. 40 year old male with aching in left arm and complaints of nausea—Priority Emergent
   b. 12 year old with cough, runny nose, and temperature 98.9 degrees F—Priority Nonurgent
   c. 42 year old female with nausea, vomiting, and abdominal pain for 3 days with temperature 105.9 degrees F—Priority Emergent
   d. 2 year old with diarrhea for 5 days, brachial pulse faintly palpable, and capillary refill time 5 seconds—Priority Urgent

3. Patients assigned an acuity rating of Urgent require:
   a. Immediate evaluation to prevent loss of life or limb
   b. Prompt care, usually within the next 1 to 2 hours
   c. Care, but time is not a critical factor in outcome

4. Reassessment in a patient with a nonurgent condition is recommended:
   a. Every 15 to 30 minutes
   b. Every 60 minutes
   c. Every 1 to 2 hours
   d. Every 8 hours

5. The triage acuity category is based on:
   a. Vital signs
   b. Clinical presentation
   c. Chief complaint
   d. All the above

6. Patients with a complaint that does not clearly fall into a specific acuity should be:
   a. Assessed by the nurse in the treatment area who will assign acuity
   b. Assigned the higher acuity that may apply to the patient
   c. Assigned all acuity levels that may apply
   d. Reassessed after 5 minutes to determine acuity

1. What type of triage system is used in your ED?
   a. Type I: Traffic director
   b. Type II: Spot-check triage
   c. Type III: Comprehensive triage
   d. Other _______________________________________

2. Diagram the triage process for your ED—from arrival at the triage desk to completion of the triage process.

3. Diagram the patient's movement through the triage process from arrival to placement in a treatment area.

Triage Assessment *chapter 2*

OBJECTIVES

After completing this chapter, you will be able to:

1. Describe four components of ED triage assessment.

2. Identify abnormal history and physical findings in the triage setting.

3. Describe history and physical findings indicating the need for emergent or urgent care.

RESOURCES

- Policies related to vital signs, pediatric triage, geriatric triage, assessment guidelines, and reassessment in the waiting area

- Diagram showing steps in the triage process for the department

- Pediatric vital sign charts with normal and abnormal ranges

- Chart showing average height and weight range for pediatric patients

INTRODUCTION

Assessment is the foundation of the nursing process and is essential for clinical decision making. Data obtained can significantly affect outcome of care. Triage assessment drives the critical triage decision. The goals of triage assessment are to identify life-threatening conditions and determine acuity level for each patient. Assessment should be done by an appropriately trained health care professional who can rapidly obtain essential data and make an appropriate determination of acuity.

The triage nurse is also the patient's first contact with the department and the facility. This contact sets the tone for communication and patient perceptions throughout the ED visit.

TRIAGE PROCESS

The process of triage is used to establish priorities and determine urgency of need for emergency care. Aspects of scientific method, diagnostic reasoning, critical thinking, personal style, and the art of nursing are found in the triage process. The triage nurse does not attempt to determine the medical diagnosis but evaluates patient condition and potential for decompensation or deterioration based on subjective, objective, historical, and physical data. This information is obtained by systematically approaching the patient within the context of the patient's current situation. Triage has four basic components: across-the-room assessment, triage history, triage physical assessment, and the triage decision. This process should take 3 to 5 minutes for most patients. Each component is addressed separately; in reality, the triage nurse may need to simultaneously perform different components for multiple patients.

Across-the-Room Assessment

Triage begins when the patient enters the triage area. With this first visual contact, the triage nurse quickly evaluates the patient's general appearance for problems that require immediate attention. This rapid assessment includes *airway, breathing, circulation,* and *disability* or neurologic status—the ABCDs of across-the-room assessment. Acuity category may be assigned at this time if the triage nurse immediately identifies an emergent life-threatening condition. Further assessment does not proceed until the patient receives appropriate treatment. Some patients may require extensive subjective and objective assessment to determine acuity.

The patient's general appearance and ABCD parameters are assessed on initial contact and with each interaction. Any significant deviation from normal requires immediate intervention. Table 2-1 lists across-the-room findings that indicate emergent problems. As you begin to observe the patient, use your eyes, ears, and nose to obtain data about the ABCDs.

General appearance: Does the patient look ill or toxic? Are posture and gait appropriate? Is the patient walking in a natural manner? Can the patient stand without assistance? Does the patient clutch any part of the body? What is the patient's skin color and facial expression? Does the patient appear angry, confused, fearful, or in pain? How does the patient interact with others and the environment?

Airway: Do you hear abnormal breathing such as stridor or wheezing? Are there signs of airway obstruction? Do you hear high-pitched sounds or barking? Is there a cough? Is breathing labored?

Circulation: What is the skin color? Is the patient pale, dusky, ashen, gray, flushed, sallow, or jaundiced? Do you see obvious bleeding?

Disability: Does the patient appear alert or sleepy? Irritable or angry? Can the patient stand and walk erect without assistance? Does the patient respond appropriately to stimulation? Does the patient appear limp or stiff? Is there obvious seizure activity?

> **Key Concept**
> Never assume that alterations in the across-the-room assessment are not life-threatening. If abnormalities are identified, act immediately. Remember, if the patient looks sick, he or she probably is (Rice & Abel, 1992).

The across-the-room assessment is the first decision point for identifying obvious life-threatening conditions. This assessment may be performed on an individual or on several patients simultaneously entering the triage area. The triage nurse can adjust the pace of the triage process to accommodate variations in flow into the triage area through use of the across-the-room assessment. This assessment is also used to scan the waiting area and quickly survey new arrivals while interviewing other patients. Should any patient appear in distress or trigger the triage nurse's antennae for trouble, the nurse can interrupt the interview and investigate.

Table 2-1. Across-the-Room Findings That Indicate Emergent Conditions	
Assessment Parameters	**Critical Findings**
Airway	•Abnormal airway sounds (e.g., stridor, wheezing, grunting) •Unusual posture (e.g., tripod or sniffing position) •Inability to speak •Drooling or inability to handle secretions
Breathing	•Altered skin signs (e.g., cyanosis, dusky skin) •Tachypnea, bradypnea, or apneic periods •Retractions •Accessory muscle use •Nasal flaring •Expiratory grunting •Prolonged expiration with pursed lips •Audible wheezes
Circulation	•Altered skin signs (e.g., pallor, mottling, flushing) •Obvious uncontrolled bleeding
Disability	•Altered level of consciousness •Decreased interaction with the environment •Inability to recognize familiar people •Unusual irritability •Decreased response to pain or stimuli •Flaccid or hyperactive muscle tone •Obvious seizure activity

TRIAGE HISTORY AND PHYSICAL ASSESSMENT

Triage begins with the across-the-room assessment and builds from that point as more information is collected. The triage history is obtained, and triage physical assessment is completed. Subjective and objective data are used during this part of the triage process. Elements are often obtained concurrently but are presented separately for training purposes.

Subjective Assessment

The patient's chief complaint, description of symptoms, and history are all subjective data obtained during triage. Collecting this data requires a common language. If the patient does not speak English or is hearing-impaired, an appropriate interpreter should be used.

Chief complaint: The chief complaint is a one-line statement in the patient's own words describing the reason for seeking emergency care. It may be necessary to ask the patient with multiple complaints to narrow the problem down to the main reason or most urgent problem that prompted the visit. Even if the complaint is vague or seemingly insignificant, remain open to the possibility that an emergency condition may be present. Think of yourself as a detective who gathers as much information as necessary to make the right decision.

Determining chief complaint is the first step in obtaining an adequate patient history. While asking questions is a good time to assess the patient for a medical alert bracelet or necklace. Questions to determine chief complaint should be asked in a friendly, professional manner. Initial questions should be open-ended statements. Asking the right question is not as easy as it sounds. Everyone hears and responds to questions differently. Questions that begin with "Why" may sound accusatory and set the wrong tone for the visit. Also, asking "What brought you today?" may prompt the patient to give you information about transportation. Individuals who are very literal may think you are truly interested in their method of transportation. The following questions are more effective:

- May I help you?

- What can we do for you?

- What is the matter?

- What is the reason you need to see the doctor today?

Once the chief complaint has been determined, the triage nurse completes a focused assessment. Always address the patient first. Acknowledge children and address appropriate questions to them. If the patient is unable to communicate, information may be provided by significant others, bystanders, or EMS personnel. Use open-ended statements during the focused assessment to allow the patient to describe symptoms. Lead the patient carefully. For example, after asking a patient to describe his back pain, ask if he or she notices anything else rather than initially offering a list of neurologic symptoms. Ask very specific questions when the patient cannot describe the problem. Notice how the patient answers questions. This can be as telling as the actual answers.

Key Concept
The patient does not have to prove he or she is sick. You as the triage nurse must prove the patient is not sick. Consider the worst-case scenario associated with that complaint, complete the assessment, and make the decision based on your assessment, not assumptions (Turner, 1981).

Presenting event: The chief complaint triggers assessment of the patient's primary concern or problem. Subjective information includes:

- Precipitating event and timing of symptom onset

- Location of the problem

- Description of the problem (e.g., nature, character, quality, severity, effect on the patient)

- Mechanism of injury, if applicable

- Progression of symptoms from onset to arrival

- Treatment prior to arrival and response to that treatment

Pain assessment: Pain is one of the most common reasons for seeking emergency care. What makes assessment of pain particularly difficult is that pain is a subjective experience that is unique for each individual. Despite these aspects of subjectivity, the triage nurse must pursue any complaint of pain. Acknowledging the patient's pain through assessment is an initial building block in the development of trust between the patient and ED staff. And remember that the patient (rather than the caregiver) determines severity of pain. A systematic approach to pain is the "PQRST" system, a rapid, effective technique to determine pain level (see Table 2-2). Patients with neuropathy or altered mental status may have increased tolerance for pain or decreased pain perception. Children have an altogether different language when it comes to pain. Findings of pain assessment contribute enormously to the triage decision. Use the Pain Scale (0 to 10) (see Fig 2-1) for adults and the Faces Scale (see Fig 2-1) for children.

Table 2-2. PQRST System of Pain Assessment

	Parameter	Assessment
P	Provokes/palliates	•What precipitated the pain? •What makes it better or worse? •What were you doing when it started?
Q	Quality	•Describe the quality of the pain. •What does it feel like?
R	Region or radiation	•Where is the pain? •How large an area is involved? •Does the pain go anywhere? Where?
S	Severity/associated symptoms	•How severe is the pain? •Rate the pain from 0 to 10 with 0 indicating no pain and 10 indicating the worst pain possible. •Do you have other problems or symptoms?
T	Timing or temporal relations	•When did the pain or symptoms start? •Is the pain constant? Does it come and go?

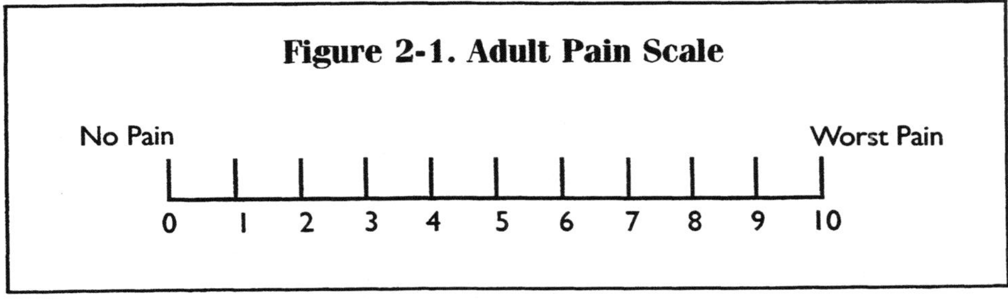

Figure 2-1. Adult Pain Scale

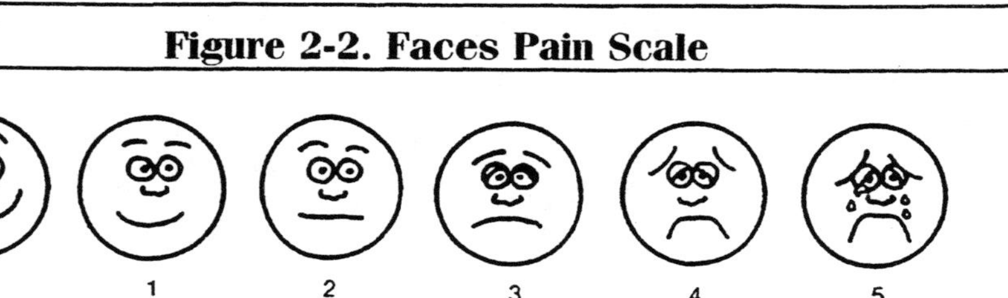

Figure 2-2. Faces Pain Scale

Associated symptoms: Once the triage nurse obtains information about the present illness and pain assessment, the patient is assessed for associated symptoms. Determining specific positive or negative information is necessary for making the triage decision. For example, the patient with lower abdominal pain who also has rectal bleeding is more severe than the patient with lower abdominal pain who complains of constipation. Open-ended questions are again used to obtain this type of information.

History: Historical information adds depth to other subjective data. Patients with certain complaints receive a greater acuity level if they also have certain medical conditions. For example, the patient with a history of hemophilia who comes to the ED with a swollen knee requires more immediate care than another patient with a swollen knee without significant medical history. The "AMPLE" mnemonic is a simple, yet systematic way to ascertain essential historical information (see Table 2-3).

Patients may underestimate the importance of medications and medical problems so the triage nurse must be alert. Routine medications, daily medications, or medications taken for minor problems such as insulin, birth control pills, or over-the-counter medications may be forgotten. Antacids or analgesics may not be mentioned unless the triage nurse specifically asks. With increasing interest in alternative therapies, many patients are using herbs and other non-traditional treatment options. Culture and religion may also determine treatment regimen so ask cultural or religious practices when appropriate.

Table 2-3. AMPLE Mnemonic for Patient History

Parameters		Description, Items, and Content
A	Allergies Age of patient	•Medications, foods, environment, latex. Describe allergic reactions when appropriate
M	Medications	•Dosage, compliance, recent changes in regimen •Over-the-counter, herbal, and home remedies
P	Past history	•Medical, surgical, pregnancy •Perinatal history for infants and children
L	Last . . .	•Last meal •Last tetanus injection and immunization status •Last menstrual period
E	Events	•What events led to this illness or injury?

Investigate medication allergies because the patient may erroneously report side effects (e.g., nausea) as an allergy. When the patient says they are allergic to anything, ask what happens when they come in contact with the suspected allergen. Ascertain specific symptoms and severity of symptoms caused by the medication. Because few EDs are latex-free, the triage nurse must also be alert to hazards posed for patients with latex allergy.

The foundation of the present is in the past. With the exception of injury, the patient's problem usually develops over time. An accurate, thorough history and physical assessment assist in making the triage decision and provide essential information for subsequent caregivers. This information helps organize the patient's care as well as ensures placement in the appropriate treatment area. For example, females with lower abdominal pain can be placed in a room equipped with a pelvic exam table.

Key Concept
Past medical and surgical events can relate to the current problem. Ascertain current medications and historical information on all patients. Document obstetrical and prenatal history when appropriate.

As you assess patient history, inquire about regular medical visits, chiropractic treatments, and previous hospitalizations. Identify risk factors and lifestyle behaviors that may contribute to the patient's primary complaint or problem. The presence of alcohol or drugs and use of cigarettes or exposure to toxic substances may be pertinent to the patient's problem and change your triage decision.

Objective Assessment

The triage nurse must assess and prioritize patients within a limited time frame. Always consider that the patient's condition can be serious or even life-threatening. Do not guess or make assumptions about the nature of the problem. Physical evaluation provides objective data about the patient's condition to assist in the triage decision. Observations such as appearance, measured data such as vital signs, and discerned data from localized examination are all part of the objective patient assessment. In order to accomplish this quickly and effectively, the triage nurse should follow a few simple steps:

- Visualize the area of complaint whenever possible. Unwrap dressings applied prior to arrival. Have the patient point with one finger to the area that is most painful.

- Compare assessment findings with the patient's baseline. Do a bilateral comparison when appropriate.

- When in doubt, check it out. Ask the patient if what you see is normal.

- Move from the least invasive or painful assessment to the most invasive or painful assessment.

Collect objective data from the body system related to the patient's chief complaint and then move to other systems as appropriate. Remember that body systems do not function independently. A problem in one system can affect other systems, just as pain from one organ may be referred to other areas of the body. Consider the patient who presents with swollen feet secondary to right-sided heart failure or the patient with a myocardial infarction whose only complaint is jaw pain. Knowledge of normal vital signs and other physical assessment parameters is essential if the triage nurse is to identify potentially serious deviations. These findings vary with age and conditions, so the triage nurse should have access to reference guides.

Focused physical assessment: A systematic approach to physical assessment using the ABCs is a simple yet effective way to assess any patients. These parameters are the same as those obtained during the across-the-room assessment; however, the depth of assessment is expanded. The initial across-the-room assessment primarily involves visualizing and listening from a distance. The focused physical assessment involves inspection, auscultation, and palpation. Percussion is rarely used in triage. Background noise and limited ability to expose various areas of the body make it difficult to obtain valid information through percussion. Table 2-4 summarizes the ABCs of focused physical assessment (ENA, 2000).

<table>
<tr><td colspan="2">Table 2-4. ABCs of the Focused Physical Assessment</td></tr>
<tr><td>Subject</td><td>Emergent or Urgent Findings</td></tr>
<tr><td>Airway</td><td>

•Abnormal airway sounds (e.g., stridor, wheezing, grunting)
•Abnormal preferred posture (e.g., tripod or sniffing position)
•Inability to speak
•Drooling or inability to handle secretions
•Dysphagia
•Abnormal breathing pattern</td></tr>
<tr><td>Breathing</td><td>

•Cool, diaphoretic, cyanotic, or dusky skin
•Tachypnea, bradypnea, or apneic periods
•Retractions
•Accessory muscle use
•Nasal flaring
•Expiratory grunting
•Prolonged expiration with pursed lips
•Diminished or absent breath sounds
•Adventitious breath sounds (e.g., crackles, wheezes, rubs)</td></tr>
<tr><td>Circulation</td><td>

•Tachycardia, bradycardia, irregular pulse, pulselessness
•Cool or hot, diaphoretic, pale, mottled, or flushed skin
•Pale mucous membranes or cyanotic nailbeds
•Delayed capillary refill
•Diminished pulse quality
•Hypotension
•Muffled, distant, variable, or adventitious heart sounds
•Obvious bleeding</td></tr>
<tr><td>Disability</td><td>

•Altered level of consciousness
•Decreased Glasgow Coma Scale
•Decreased interaction with the environment
•Inability to recognize familiar people
•Unusual irritability
•Decreased response to pain
•Flaccid or hyperactive muscle tone
•Unequal, nonreactive, or misshapen pupils
•Seizure activity</td></tr>
<tr><td>Expose</td><td>

•Asymmetry of chest or abdomen
•Extremity deformities
•Unusual or severe bruising
•Petechiae or purpura
•Uncontrolled bleeding</td></tr>
<tr><td>Full vital signs</td><td>

•Temperature, pulse rate, respiratory rate, and blood pressure
•Decreased oxygen saturation
•Decreased BP or increased pulse with orthostatic vital sign assessment
•Asymmetrical BP and/or pulse</td></tr>
<tr><td>G</td><td>

•Give comfort measures—reassurance, touch, pain control</td></tr>
<tr><td>Head-to-toe history</td><td>

•Additional injuries, abnormalities, or areas of tenderness, discoloration, or bruising</td></tr>
</table>

Adapted from Emergency Nurses Association (ENA). (2000). *Trauma nursing core curriculum* [Provider Manual] (5th ed.). Des Plaines, IL: Author. p 313-314.

The Glasgow Coma Scale is used for baseline neurologic assessment and monitoring trends over time. The score provides limited information, but has been used as a predictor of outcome in trauma patients.

Figure 2-2. Glasgow Coma Scale Score

Areas of Response	Points
Best Eye Opening	
Eyes open spontaneously	4
Eyes open in response to voice	3
Eyes open in response to pain	2
No eye opening response	1
Best Verbal Response	
Oriented (e.g., to person, place, time)	5
Confused, speaks but is disoriented	4
Inappropriate, but comprehensible words	3
Incomprehensible sounds but no words are spoken	2
None	1
Best Motor Response	
Obeys command to move	6
Localizes painful stimulus	5
Withdraws from painful stimulus	4
Flexion, abnormal decorticate posturing	3
Extension, abnormal decerebrate posturing	2
No movement or posturing	1
Total Possible Points	**3-15**
Severe Head Injury	**<8**
Moderate Head Injury	**9-12**
Minor Head Injury	**13-15**

Adequate assessment requires visual and tactile assessment; therefore, areas of concern should be exposed and examined. Maintain patient privacy during these examinations and use universal precautions. If an area cannot be exposed in the triage area, elicit as much information as possible from the patient regarding the problem. Once the patient is placed in a treatment area, the area can be exposed and assessment completed. The area of concern may be left uncovered to facilitate continued assessment. This is particularly effective for extremities. Touch the patient to determine skin temperature and presence of moisture. A simple touch can provide a wealth of information and help to reassure the patient. Be sure to maintain the patient's body heat, particularly for pediatric and geriatric patients. Infants are often bundled in numerous clothes and blankets—even those with fevers. Remove clothes to allow the heat to dissipate.

Key Concept
Touch the patient to ascertain skin temperature, presence of moisture, and presence of an irregular pulse.

Vital signs provide essential information about the patient's condition. Noninvasive blood pressure (NIBP) monitors are frequently used in triage areas. Manual readings should be obtained when monitor readings are suspicious or numbers do not correlate to clinical exam. These machines do not detect pulse irregularities, so the triage nurse should palpate the pulse when a dysrhythmia is suspected. Obtaining vital signs in children requires patience and skill. Machines can frighten children and make the process more difficult. Begin with the least invasive test and move to the most invasive. For example, observe respirations first, then heart rate, and, finally, temperature.

> **Key Concept**
> **Obtain manual blood pressure when NIBP numbers are suspicious or significantly abnormal.**

AGE-RELATED CONSIDERATIONS

Some EDs specialize in treating children; however, none are uniquely dedicated to care of elderly patients. Geography and demographics are more indicative of age groups a given ED will see. In general, emergency nurses and most EDs care for patients of all ages. Despite similarities in process, assessment and treatment of pediatric and geriatric groups vary significantly from each other and from the usual adult ED patient. The triage nurse must not only be familiar with the predominant age groups seen in the facility's ED, but also be prepared to assess and treat infants, children, and elderly patients. Elder and pediatric patients are the populations most at risk for abuse and neglect. Chapter 11: Abuse and Neglect discusses how to assess abuse in these and other patient groups.

Pediatric Patients

Children are definitely not small adults. Variations in vital signs, anatomy, physiology, and psychosocial constructs make triage and treatment of pediatric patients a challenge. Table 2-5 presents unique aspects of pediatric anatomy and physiology that must be considered during triage. Pediatric assessment should be tailored to the patient's developmental level and ability to communicate. The ABCD approach is used for children with special attention given to differences in this population. Table 2-6 outlines pediatric assessment and interventions using this approach.

Table 2-5. Anatomic and Physiologic Considerations in Pediatric Assessment

Parameter	Description of Variations
Airway	•Neonates are obligate nose breathers. •Airway is smaller but increases in size as the patient grows. •Tongue is larger in proportion to mouth.
Breathing	•Infants are more reliant on the diaphragm for effective ventilation. •Ribs are horizontal, soft, and cartilaginous. •Chest wall is thin and respiratory muscles are poorly developed. •Fatigue occurs quickly with respiratory distress. •Normal respiratory rates decrease as age increases. •Greater oxygen requirement because of increased basal metabolic rate (BMR).
Circulation	•Normal pulse rates decrease as age increases. •Brachial or apical sites are used for infant pulse checks. •Circulating blood volume is 85 ml/kg in neonates, 80 ml/kg in infants, and 75 ml/kg in children. •Functional murmurs are often present in infants. •Cardiac output is greatly influenced by heart rate. •Hypotension is a late sign of shock and may not appear until volume loss is 24 to 40%.
Cervical spine	•Head in infant and child is significantly larger and heavier in relation to body size. •Laxity of cervical spine ligaments, shallow facet joints, and poorly developed musculature make the cervical spine more elastic and mobile.
Disability	•Anterior fontanel normally closes at 18 to 24 months. •Pain response is expressed according to age (e.g., kicking and jerking in infants, verbalization in schoolage children).
Exposure	•Larger body surface area (BSA) to weight ratio increases ambient heat loss. •Infants cannot shiver because of neuromuscular immaturity. •Temperature control is not fully developed in infants, so hypothermia occurs more quickly.
F	•Extremities may feel cold because of peripheral vasoconstriction despite presence of high fever.
Get vital signs	•Vital signs vary significantly with age. •Sinus tachycardia is a common response to many stressors. •Bradycardia in a child is an ominous sign.

Table 2-6. ABCD Mnemonic for Pediatric Assessment

Parameter	Assessment	Intervention
Airway	•Determine patency, position, audible sounds, airway obstruction (e.g., blood, mucous, edema)	•Allow child to maintain position of comfort or position airway with jaw thrust or head tilt-chin lift •Use airway adjuncts as required
Breathing	•Observe for increased or decreased work of breathing, nasal flaring, use of accessory muscles, pattern, quality	•Provide supplemental oxygen •Initiate assisted ventilation with BVM and intubate as indicated •Provide gastric decompression with orogastric or nasogastric tube
Circulation	•Observe for skin color, capillary refill, strength of peripheral and central pulses, skin temperature, peripheral and/or central cyanosis and mottling	•Obtain vascular access •Initiate volume replacement •Perform chest compressions •Defibrillate or provide synchronized cardioversion •Initiate drug therapy
Disability	•Determine activity level, level of consciousness, response to environment, response to parent, pupillary response	•Treat underlying cause (e.g., signs of increased intracranial pressure, fluid or blood loss, hypoxia)
Expose	•Identify underlying injuries or other signs of illness	•Remove clothes, including diapers
F	•Determine core temperature •Assess for shivering	•Maintain normothermic environment •Initiate supplemental rewarming measures
Get vital signs	•Evaluate temperature, pulse and respirations, BP as appropriate, weight in kilograms	•Continuously monitor vital signs •Obtain weight estimate if condition does not permit measured weight
Head-to-toe history	•Perform complete head-to-toe assessment and history, including immunizations, and assess for unusual odors	•Continuously monitor child for changes in condition
Inspect back; isolate	•Observe back for obvious or hidden injuries and assess for communicable illness or susceptibility to illness such as in an immune-suppressed patient	•Reassess back as indicated •Isolate when indicated

Working with infants and children takes patience and experience. It is important to remember that parents and child should be treated as a unit. Avoid separation. Parents know their child better than anyone else. When a parent says the child is not acting right, this is essential information and should not be casually dismissed. Additionally, the child should not be ignored. Involve the child in the discussion to obtain as much information as possible. When treating children, always be honest and tell them what you are going to do and if it will hurt. Explain the procedure in terms they can understand and in ways that do not frighten them. For example, describing a little magic machine that makes noise when put in the ears and a penlight that can be blown out are less frightening than using medical terms (Magid, 1993). Children are very conscious of their bodies, and they may be very shy at certain ages. Protect their modesty and respect their privacy. As you triage the pediatric patient, also assess the parent. Consider how the parent and child interact and what stress is created by the specific situation. Consider the possibility of abuse and neglect when the patient's history does not match the physical findings. Cardinal indicators of abuse include cigarette burns, and bruises with a distinct pattern such as a belt buckle (see Chapter 11: Abuse and Neglect).

Geriatric Patients

Elderly patients are more likely to have chronic health problems that alter findings in the triage assessment and make minor problems more complicated. Anatomical and physiologic changes because of normal aging cause changes in vital signs, mobility, and perceptions. Table 2-7 presents unique aspects of geriatric anatomy and physiology that must be considered during assessment. Just as pediatric assessment is tailored to each child's developmental level and ability to communicate, geriatric assessment should also be tailored to the individual. Geriatric patients, like most adults, have their own way of doing things. Attempting to change this pattern—even in something so seemingly insignificant as how the patient removes his or her sweater—can cause resentment or confusion. Approach these patients with respect. Do not use the patient's first name unless requested to do so. Allow the patient time to answer and perform any activity.

Elderly patients may dismiss significant symptoms as a normal part of aging. Evaluate negatives as well as positives. The older patient may also be on numerous over-the-counter medications and prescription medications that are often prescribed by different providers. Document current medications including over-the-counter medications and home remedies. Substance abuse problems and depression are also found in elderly patients, so psychological assessment is important. As you care for the elderly patient, remember that physiologic changes in the skin make it easy to injure the skin. Applying a tourniquet or holding the patient firmly can bruise or even tear fragile skin. Assess skin before you touch the patient.

Table 2-7. Geriatric Assessment Overview

Parameter	Variation/Description
Airway	•Diminished sense of smell •Increased likelihood of posterior nosebleeds •Diminished protective mechanisms
Breathing	•Decreased elasticity in small airways •Decreased vital capacity •Limited chest wall expansion •Barrel chest appearance •Lower oxygen saturation and tension •Decreased resistance to infection
Circulation	•Decreased cardiac reserve •Slight decrease in heart rate •Slowed, decreased response to stress •Stiffened arterial walls, so BP increases, upper pulses are more pronounced, and pedal pulses may not be detected •Increased likelihood of inflammation and varicosity because veins become tortuous
Cervical spine	•Decreased bone mass •Joint erosion •Loss of muscle mass •Loss of elasticity in ligaments and cartilage
Disability	•Decreased cerebral blood flow •Decreased number of functioning neurons •Decreased transmission velocity •Diminished short-term memory •Depressed sense of pain •Decreased pupillary response and accommodation
Exposure	•Decreased subcutaneous fat •Decreased extracellular water •Diminished blood supply •Thinning outer skin layers and thickened nails
F	•Decreased efficiency of temperature regulation •Slowed sensory perceptions
Get vital signs	•Potential for orthostatic changes because of changes in aging or effects of medication •Asymmetrical BP values, which may be due to changes with aging or secondary to aortic dissection or aneurysm

TRIAGE DECISION

The triage decision is the culmination of a complex process based on assessment of the patient's condition, potential for deterioration within various time frames, and availability of resources. Table 2-8 reviews processes used to reach the triage decision. These steps may be done consecutively or simultaneously for one or many patients; however, the importance of each step should not be minimized. The triage decision is not set in stone; in fact, it changes when patient acuity changes. Once the triage decision is made and acuity is determined, any qualifiers should be identified so the patient can be placed in the appropriate treatment area. For example, the patient with severe migraine pain benefits from a quiet, dimly lit room, whereas a patient with ocular burns may be placed in a special "eye" room. As the triage nurse gains experience, his or her assessment style and critical thinking skills improve and the process becomes streamlined.

> **Key Concept**
> Discontinue assessment and transport the patient immediately to the treatment area if immediate care is needed. Do not delay treatment to finish the assessment.

Table 2-8. Systematic Triage Decision Process

Step 1	Observe the patient. Perform visual survey.
Step 2	Determine chief complaint and perform primary survey.
Step 3	Perform focused assessment of chief complaint, obtain subjective assessment related to present condition, and complete objective assessment.
Step 4	Consider "worst-case scenarios," pose hypotheses, and collect data to narrow the range of possibilities. Consider current condition, potential for deterioration, speed of flow within the department, and resource availability.
Step 5	Determine acuity category (i.e., make the triage decision).
Step 6	Reassess and reassign acuity as necessary.

REASSESSMENT

When treatment space is not immediately available, patients with lower acuity remain in the waiting area. These patients are reassessed at periodic intervals to ensure that no change in acuity has occurred. Reassessment is based on the patient's initial assessment and acuity determination. Specifics of reassessment include, but are not limited to, repeat vital signs and focused assessment. Significant symptoms are reassessed to determine if the condition has improved or worsened. Patients may also be visually assessed each time the triage nurse observes the waiting area. The triage nurse should advise the patient to return to the triage area if symptoms worsen or if any change occurs that concerns the patient.

> **Key Concept**
> If the patient's condition changes, reassess to determine if the patient requires more immediate attention.

SUMMARY

The triage nurse is challenged to obtain concise, useful subjective and objective data in a small amount of time while maintaining vigilance over patients who are waiting and arriving. The effective triage nurse uses a systematic approach to focus assessment on the specific problem while remaining flexible to accommodate the unexpected.

References

Emergency Nurses Association. (2000). <u>Trauma nursing core curriculum</u> [Provider Manual] (5th ed.). Des Plaines, IL: Author.

Emergency Nurses Association. (1997). <u>Triage: Meeting the challenge.</u> (2nd ed.). Park Ridge, IL: Author.

Emergency Nurses Association. (1998). <u>Emergency nursing pediatric course</u> [Provider Manual] (2nd ed.). Park Ridge, IL: Author.

Emergency Nurses Association. (1992). <u>Triage: Meeting the challenge.</u> Chicago: Author.

Jordan, K. (Ed.). (2000). <u>Emergency nursing core curriculum</u> (5th ed.). Philadelphia: Saunders.

Kellett, P.B. (1997). Latex allergy: A review. <u>Journal of Emergency Nursing, 23</u>(2), 27-36.

Kidd, P., & Sturt, P. (1996). <u>Mosby's emergency nursing reference.</u> St. Louis: Mosby.

Kitt, S., Selfridge-Thomas, J., Proehl, J., & Kaiser, K. (1995). <u>Emergency nursing: A physiologic and clinical perspective</u> (2nd ed.). Philadelphia: Saunders

Lewis, S.M., Collier, I.C., & Heitkemper, M.M. (1999). <u>Medical-surgical nursing: Assessment and management of clinical problems</u> (5th ed.). St. Louis: Mosby.

Magid, E. (1993). Pediatric triage. <u>The Monitor, 1</u>(4), 3.

McCaffery, M. (1968). <u>Cognition, bodily pain and man-environment interactions.</u> Los Angeles: University of California.

Neff, J., & Kidd, P. (1993). <u>Trauma nursing: The art and science.</u> St. Louis: Mosby.

Newberry, L. (1998). <u>Sheehy's emergency nursing: Principles and practice</u> (4th ed.). St. Louis: Mosby.

Rice, M., & Abel, C. (1992). In S. Budassi-Sheehy (Ed.)., <u>Emergency nursing: Principles and practice</u> (3rd ed.). St. Louis: Mosby-Year Book.

Turner, S.R. (1981). Golden rules for accurate triage. <u>Journal of Emergency Nursing, 7</u>(4), 153.

Wolf, A. (1998). Latex allergy: Relevant to us all. <u>American Journal of Nursing, 98</u>(3), 80.

1. Which of the following statements is most effective in obtaining information about the patient's chief complaint?
   a. Are you having chest pain?
   b. Do you have any medical problems that we need to know about?
   c. What brought you to the ED today?
   d. Why do you need to see the doctor today?

2. A patient with which of the following presentations should be transported immediately to the treatment area?
   a. Deformity of lower extremity after jumping from a stationary truck
   b. Stab wound to left calf with no bleeding or pain
   c. Gunshot wound to right hand 12 hours prior to arrival
   d. Pelvis crushed between truck and brick wall

3. Complete the following table on components of triage assessment.
   A = Across the room
   S = Subjective assessment
   O = Objective assessment
   F = Focused physical assessment

Component	Item
	Level of consciousness
	Precipitating event
	Quality and quantity of pain
	Allergies to drugs or latex
	Current medications
	Radial pulse rate and character
	Visual assessment of injuries
	Breathing pattern
	Evidence of bleeding
	Patient temperature

4. The initial step in the triage process is to:
   a. Determine chief complaint and complete a primary survey
   b. Observe the patient and perform a visual survey
   c. Determine triage acuity
   d. Obtain subjective and objective information about the complaint

5. Findings in the across-the-room assessment that indicate emergent conditions
include:
   a. Tachycardia
   b. Mild epistaxis
   c. Tachypnea
   d. Deformity of left forearm

6. Triage findings from the focused physical assessment that indicate an urgent or
emergent condition include:
   a. Mild, diffuse wheezing
   b. Drooling or inability to handle secretions
   c. Symmetrical blood pressure and/or pulse
   d. Facial lacerations

7. Which of the following patient situations should be triaged as emergent?
   a. Lower abdominal pain for 12 hours
   b. Needle stick from known AIDS patient
   c. Pulse oximetry 96% on room air
   d. Orthostatic pulse increases 10 points when patient stands

8. Four school-aged children are injured in a fistfight during recess. On arrival to
the ED, which child's injury is emergent?
   a. Superficial lacerations of eyebrow and face
   b. Ecchymosis and swelling of orbital area
   c. Blood in the anterior chamber
   d. Abrasions and scratches of eyes and forehead

1. Observe the triage nurse in your ED performing triage assessment on a patient with a chief complaint of pain. After completion of triage, determine if the triage assessment elicited the following components of pain assessment:

Pain Assessment	Yes	No
What precipitated the pain?		
What makes the pain better or worse?		
What were you doing when the pain started?		
Describe the quality of your pain.		
Can you tell me what how the pain feels?		
Point to the area of pain.		
How large of an area is hurting?		
Does the pain go anywhere else?		
Rate the pain on a scale from 0 to 10.		
Make a subjective rating—no pain, tolerable, moderate, severe, unbearable.		
Do you have other symptoms with this pain?		
When did the pain or these symptoms start?		
Is the pain constant or does it come and go?		

2. Identify resources available in the triage area to facilitate assessment of the pediatric patient.

OBJECTIVES

After completing this chapter, you will be able to:

1. Describe three primary goals of triage documentation.

2. Identify five essential components of triage documentation.

3. Discuss two elements of essential documentation elements for patients who leave before receiving definitive care.

RESOURCES

- Blank copy of the ED chart, nursing documentation forms, and other related documentation tools

- Policies related to ED charting, triage documentation, protocols, and patient disposition

- Examples of quality monitoring tools related to triage

INTRODUCTION

Triage documentation should support the triage decision, communicate essential information to other caregivers, and comply with regulatory and legal mandates. Your institution may require additional data. Format used by a given institution is affected by staffing patterns, patient acuity, current technology, and departmental culture. Documentation may be a handwritten narrative or a check-off format. Increased availability of computerized documentation programs has increased the number of EDs that use computers for nursing documentation. Appendix C provides samples of triage documentation tools.

Regardless of format, requirements for triage documentation are the same. Table 3-1 lists essential components for triage documentation. In addition to these components, the Joint Commission on Accreditation of Health Care Organizations (JCAHO) requires assessment of learning needs and cultural, religious, and spiritual needs related to care (JCAHO, 1998). The chart should also reflect assessment of developmental issues for pediatric patients.

Table 3-1. Essential Components of Triage Documentation

•Time seen by the triage nurse	•Chief complaint
•Allergies	•Current medications
•Vital signs	•Subjective and objective assessment
•Patient acuity rating	•Diagnostic tests and triage actions
•Disposition	•Reassessment

Triage documentation should follow the same basic principles as other nursing documentation, including legibility, appropriate signatures, correction of errors, and use of accepted medical abbreviations (Newberry, 1998). Do not chart assumptions or things you do not know. For example, the patient may smell of alcohol, but you should not chart that the patient is intoxicated if you do not know the serum ethanol level. Describe the patient's behavior without judgmental commentary.

> **Key Concept**
> **Document as if the next time you see the chart it will be in court.**

INITIAL DOCUMENTATION

Triage documentation may be done as a single step by one person, or it may be done in stages by one triage nurse or two different triage nurses. When several patients arrive at the triage area simultaneously, the triage nurse screens patients to identify those who require immediate care. This type of screening is limited to visual and verbal assessment. Tactile examination may be done on select patients; however, vital signs are usually not taken in this situation. Documentation for this type of screening includes name, chief complaint, and a brief description of appearance and patient acuity. The need for an interpreter is usually identified during the first contact with the patient. This documentation provides a "snapshot" of the patient at that point in time (Newberry, 1998). If the patient leaves before further assessment and suffers an adverse outcome, this documentation may offer the hospital some legal protection.

TIME SEEN BY TRIAGE NURSE

Document the time you begin evaluation of the patient in the triage area. Use of military time may be required by some institutions. Time of subsequent evaluations and interactions should also be documented. This documentation can provide information for caregivers and serve as a time line for the patient's visit to the ED.

CHIEF COMPLAINT

The chief complaint is written in the patient's own words using quotes as appropriate. It is also acceptable to write the complaint as a sentence fragment without quotes. For example, "I have a sprained ankle" may be written as c/o sprain ankle. The advantage of using direct quotes is that the patient's impression is clearly documented. If the patient provides specific expectations, such as "I need a shot," "I need to be admitted," or "I need an x-ray," these should also be documented. Record obstacles for communicating with the patient (e.g., language barriers, hearing limitations, mental disability).

ALLERGIES

Medication allergies should be identified and specific reactions documented. Description of the allergic response helps clarify true allergies from expected side effects such as nausea. Allergies to latex and tape should also be documented. JCAHO stresses the importance of including food allergies (1998).

MEDICATIONS

All medications the patient takes on a regular basis should be listed, including over-the-counter medications, prescription medications, and home remedies. Be sure to question the patient about medicines taken recently, such as a single dose of pain medication. Your institution may only require documentation of the drug, whereas another institution may require the triage nurse to document drug, dosage, and frequency. Patients taking multiple medications may keep a list with them that can be copied and attached to the patient chart.

VITAL SIGNS

Temperature, pulse, and respiratory rate are documented on all patients. Identify how the temperature was obtained and any irregularity of pulse or respiratory pattern. Blood pressure (BP) documentation is required for adults and children with certain complaints or clinical presentations. The age when BP is routinely obtained varies by institution, usually beginning with adolescents. Orthostatic vital signs should be documented for patients with potential volume deficits and complaints of dizziness when standing. Document BP in both arms for patients with suspected aortic disease. Other requirements may be specified by your institution.

SUBJECTIVE AND OBJECTIVE ASSESSMENT

The triage nurse must rapidly assess the patient and determine acuity. Documentation should facilitate and support this process without delaying care. A patient who is ashen, diaphoretic, and complains of chest pain requires minimal documentation by the triage nurse. Documentation of the patient's life history is not appropriate.

Key Concept
Document sufficient information to justify the triage decision.

Historical documentation varies by patient, but basic information includes current medical conditions, pertinent surgical procedures, obstetrical history, and immunization status. Date of last menstrual period and method of contraception are documented for women of reproductive age.

Other objective data that may be documented include oxygen saturation level, weight, height, and immunization status. Requirements for these vary by institution.

Subjective data should be documented carefully. Document patient denials if they conflict with objective findings or add significant information for subsequent caregivers. For example, denial of neck pain by a patient who dove into shallow water and has a laceration on the top of the head is cogent information. Another example is "multiple wrist lacerations—denies trying to kill self." In addition to documentation that a patient may be a danger to self or others, steps taken to protect the patient and others should be documented.

ACUITY CATEGORY

Most ED charts have a designated area to document acuity level. Change in acuity must be documented and include when the change occurred and the new acuity level assigned to the patient. The new acuity level may be documented in the same area as the original acuity or in another designated area. Additional information in narrative or checklist format should support any documented change in acuity.

DIAGNOSTIC TESTS AND TRIAGE ACTIONS

Document any diagnostic tests ordered at triage (e.g., lab tests, x-rays). Triage actions such as application of splints, administration of medications, and finger stick glucose testing are also documented. The patient's response to these actions should be noted.

DISPOSITION

Most EDs do not require documentation when the patient is taken from triage to the treatment area because the record of the room or bed where the patient is placed indirectly documents this. Tiered systems with different triage stations may require documentation of treatment area. Disposition of patients elsewhere must meet Emergency Medical Treatment and Active Labor Act (EMTALA) requirements for a medical screening examination (MSE). The procedure must be carefully documented and include who made the decision and how the patient will get to the intended destination. This process of "triaging out" should be guided by carefully crafted written protocols with defined sources for alternative care (Newberry, 1998).

REASSESSMENT

Reassessment is done when there is a change in the patient's condition or acuity level. Urgent patients should be reassessed every 30 to 60 minutes, whereas nonurgent patients may be reassessed every 1 to 2 hours. Your facility may have established more stringent time parameters. Carefully document changes in the patient's condition and adjust acuity level accordingly. Record actions taken when the patient's condition changes.

EMTALA CONSIDERATIONS

Patients who come to the ED must be offered an MSE before financial discussions (ENA, 1999). If the patient chooses to leave after this exam, the facility has met its obligations under EMTALA (Kadzielski & Gordon, 1998). Patients who choose to leave before the MSE should be asked to sign a form that clearly states the patient was offered an MSE, was not denied emergency care, and chooses to seek care elsewhere. Requirements for a MSE do not vary from state to state—EMTALA is federal legislation. Patients cannot be refused care; however, insurance companies can refuse to pay for this care. This has created confusion for the public and for many health care providers. (Refer to Chapter 4: Legal Issues for more discussion of EMTALA.)

Patients may also walk out without notice before the MSE. The triage nurse may be required to document this on a special "left before seen" form or in the triage record. Carefully document when you noticed the patient was gone and what efforts you made to find the patient. Record telephone calls made to the patient's home or law enforcement. The facility may also require the triage nurse to complete an incident report. If so, care should be taken that the incident report is not mentioned in the medical record.

SUMMARY

Triage documentation provides information to subsequent caregivers as well as protects the triage nurse. Appropriate triage documentation supports decisions made by the triage nurse and shows adherence to institutional policies and procedures. The challenge for the triage nurse is to document quickly without loss of quality.

References

Joint Commission on Accreditation of Healthcare Organizations (JCAHO). (1998). <u>Comprehensive accreditation manual for hospitals: The official handbook</u>. Chicago: Author.

Jordan, K. (Ed.). (2000). <u>Emergency nursing core curriculum</u> (5th ed.). Philadelphia: Saunders.

Kadzielski, M., & Gordon, J. (1998, September). COBRA's bite: Is it getting worse? An analysis of HCFA'S guidelines on patient dumping. <u>Hospital Outlook</u>, 6-7.

Newberry, L. (Ed.). (1998). *Sheehy's emergency nursing: Principles and practice* (4th ed.). St. Louis: Mosby.

1. Essential documentation by the triage nurse includes:
   a. Acuity rating
   b. Vital signs
   c. Allergies
   d. All the above

2. Chief complaint should be documented:
   a. As a potential diagnosis
   b. In the patient's own words
   c. As a complete sentence
   d. Written as a system problem (e.g., respiratory problem)

3. Essential data that should be documented on patients who leave without seeing the physician include:
   a. Private physician
   b. Condition at time the patient leaves
   c. Home telephone number and address
   d. Managed care provider

4. Which of the following statements is NOT true about triage documentation?
   a. Documentation should support the acuity assigned to the patient.
   b. Information must be documented exactly the same for all patients regardless of complaint.
   c. Documentation may be handwritten or done by computer.
   d. Documentation should communicate essential information to other caregivers.

5. Joint Commission on Accreditation of Healthcare Organizations requires that which of the following is assessed on all patients?
   a. Height
   b. Head circumference
   c. Religious needs
   d. Previous surgeries

6. Pertinent historical information for the patient who presents with an open fracture of the left forearm includes:
   a. Cholecystectomy 3 years ago
   b. Family history of cardiac disease
   c. Receiving chemotherapy for Hodgkins Lymphoma
   d. Fracture right ankle 10 years ago

7. Orthostatic vital signs should be documented on which of the following patients?
   a. 57 year old female sent from the health department with high blood pressure
   b. 24 year old female with nausea and vomiting for three days
   c. 44 year old female with intermittent dizziness for one year
   d. 36 year old female with acute onset left flank pain

1. Describe the acuity system used in your ED and provide examples for each level.

2. Identify triage documentation standards used in your facility.

3. Review triage documentation tools used in your facility.

4. Discuss the importance of obtaining the patient's medication history at triage.

5. Review the importance of documenting the patient's time of arrival, time of onset of injury or illness, and time of patient recheck.

6. Identify mandatory documentation requirements for triage.

Legal Issues *chapter 4*

OBJECTIVES

After completing this chapter, you will be able to:

1. Discuss three legal concerns related to triage.

2. Identify two resources available to the triage nurse when legal questions arise.

3. Define the triage nurse's responsibility regarding patients with hearing impairments.

RESOURCES

- Policies related to Emergency Medical Treatment and Active Labor Act (EMTALA), release of medical records, consent for treatment, holding patients against their will, confidentiality, telephone advice, leaving against medical advice (AMA), refusing treatment, restraints, American Disabilities Act (ADA)

- Policies related to reportable patient situations, legal blood and urine collection, evidence collection, and chain of custody

- Policies related to advance directives, living wills, and durable powers of attorney

INTRODUCTION

Multiple, complex legal issues affect triage. Changes in state and federal laws from new case law interpretation challenge the triage nurse to remain current in applicable legal issues. In addition to state and federal laws, institutions may have more stringent interpretations of specific regulations. The most common legal issues are described in this chapter; however, this information is offered as a review only. Study pertinent institutional policies for specifics that apply to practice in your department and state.

CONSENT

Written consent for treatment is required unless the patient is physically or mentally unable to provide it. The age at which a patient can give consent varies from state to state—as young as 14 years up to 18 years. The patient's spouse, parent, or adult child can give *involuntary consent* when the patient cannot. Laws vary from state to state; however, those listed in Table 4-1 are generally allowed to give consent. These are listed in order of priority for giving consent. Consent for treatment covers assessment, evaluation, diagnostic tests such as lab and x-ray, and other treatments. It does not cover surgical procedures and invasive diagnostic procedures. Implied consent allows treatment in emergency situations under the premise that the patient would give consent if able to do so (ENA, 1999; Kitt, Selfridge-Thomas, Proehl, & Kaiser, 1995; Newberry, 1998).

Table 4-1. Individuals Who Can Give Involuntary Consent
•Spouse who is legally married
•Spouse who is common law
•Parent
•Adult child
•Adult sibling
•Adult aunt, uncle, or grandparent
•Court system
(ENA, 1997)

Most states allow pregnant women of any age to consent to treatment. Emancipated minors (i.e., individuals below the age of consent who are self-supporting and recognized in a legal capacity as an adult) are also recognized in most states. Consent for other minors must come from a legal guardian unless the physician determines the patient requires emergency treatment to prevent significant morbidity or loss of life.

> **Key Concept**
> **Consent for treatment must be obtained for any minor that is not emancipated. If a parent or guardian cannot be reached, the physician should examine the patient to rule out an emergent condition.**

MEDICAL RECORD

The medical record is a legal document that describes the patient's care. The record reflects the sequence of events that occurred during the time the patient spent in the facility. Lab results and x-rays are considered part of the medical record. A paper record is most common, but more and more facilities are moving toward computerized documentation.

The triage note provides information about presenting complaint and a description of patient status on arrival. A precise description at this point is critical if the patient leaves before a medical screening examination (MSE) is done.

Laws governing release of patient records vary from state to state; however, usual practice is that records are not released without written consent from the patient or an authorized representative. Copies of records may be mailed, picked up, or sent by fax machine. Fax transmittal of mental health records and physician orders is not the usual practice—refer to institutional polices regarding release and/or fax transmittal of these and other patient records. Original x-rays are usually released for critical patients after final interpretation by a radiologist. Some institutions release copies rather than risk loss of original films.

CONFIDENTIALITY

The patient has a right to privacy and confidentiality. Personal information is shared only with those involved in care. This applies to written, verbal, and computerized data. The triage area is usually an open area, so privacy and confidentiality can be a challenge. Be sensitive—the patient may not wish to explain his or her problem in this open, exposed area. Whenever possible, provide visual and verbal privacy. Monitor the volume of your voice during interviews to ensure that others in the waiting area cannot hear.

Busy EDs often receive inquiries about accident victims or shooting victims. Each state has laws regarding release of information about these and other patient situations. Many facilities designate certain patients as "no information" (e.g., mental health admissions, celebrities, patients in protective custody). Check the computer or facility log to determine if information can be released about a specific patient. When you are not sure, err on the side of confidentiality.

The ED by its very nature attracts the media. Events such as shootings, car accidents, and outbreaks of meningitis are a source of news for the press. Your facility may have media representatives who provide interviews, answer questions, and run interference. When media support is not available, problems with release of information and crowd control may develop. Anyone charged with interacting with the media should be familiar with the facility's policies regarding release of information as well as definitions for critical, serious, fair, and stable conditions. Policies usually discuss filming in parking lots, waiting rooms, and treatment areas. Become familiar with these policies and know whom to call when reporters do not comply with written expectations.

Many EDs have special behavior control rooms equipped with observation windows and cameras. Be very careful when these rooms are used for patients who do not require mental health observation or seclusion. Camera observation is appropriate for the patient placed in seclusion, but should never be used without a seclusion order. The reason for seclusion and mandatory observation should be documented on a seclusion-monitoring sheet. Camera monitors should be placed to ensure the confidentiality of patients who are being monitored.

State law requires mandatory reporting of certain crimes and situations (e.g., gunshot wounds, child abuse, and neglect). Other situations may not be so clear cut. For example, should you report the patient who possesses an illegal substance or the intoxicated patient who insists on driving home? These situations may be addressed by state law or department policy. Check with your facility's risk management department for additional information.

TELEPHONE ADVICE

Patients frequently call the ED for information and advice, and many of the calls come to the triage nurse. These calls are fraught with danger for the nurse who does not follow department policy. The patient may not have given the nurse important medical information or may not understand the directions given by the nurse. This type of confusion can lead to potentially lethal situations. For example, a mother who is directed to place her child with a fever in a tub of tepid water may leave the child unattended. The child may have a febrile seizure and drown in the tub. The safest approach to these calls is to direct the person to seek emergency care.

Some EDs do provide advice over the telephone. When telephone advice is given, the nurse should follow established protocols. Unfortunately, even use of rigid protocols does not ensure consistent advice for callers (Mitchell, 1999). Ideally, telephone advice is provided with very specific protocols, each call is logged, and follow-up calls are made to determine patient condition. Consult your department policy for specific guidelines.

Emergency Medical Treatment and Active Labor Act (EMTALA)

The EMTALA of 1986—part of the Consolidated Omnibus Reconciliation Act (COBRA) of the same year—was the legislature's answer to "patient dumping." EMTALA requires that anyone seeking emergency care be offered a medical screening examination (MSE) to rule out an emergent medical condition. The MSE must take place before discussion of finances (ENA, 1999). There has been some controversy about what constitutes the MSE and who should perform it. Your facility's bylaws must specify who can perform the MSE.

Medical Screening Examination (MSE)

Triage does not fulfill the legal definition of MSE. The MSE is a "process required to reach with reasonable clinical confidence, the point at which it can be determined whether a medical emergency does or does not exist" (Health Care Financing Administration [HCFA], 1998). The MSE begins at triage but is not completed until an emergent medical condition is ruled out. In the past, physicians, physician assistants, nurse practitioners, or nurses have done the MSE. However, as the definition for MSE becomes broader and more inclusive, it is more appropriate to limit the MSE to physicians or physician extenders such as nurse practitioners or physician assistants. Delegating the MSE to the triage nurse is fraught with risk and is not encouraged.

The next issue related to the MSE is financial. Any institution that asks financial questions or collects the insurance co-pay before the MSE has committed an EMTALA violation. Institutions are investigating ways to meet these requirements while still remaining financially sound. Completing registration after the physician visit or at the end of the visit are two options. Regardless of how this is done at your facility, focus on the patient before you focus on the finances.

Emergent Medical Condition

The definition of what constitutes an emergency varies. The patient may have an entirely different definition than the health care provider. For legal purposes, EMTALA specifically defines an emergent medical condition as "Acute symptoms of sufficient severity including pain that the absence of immediate medical attention could be reasonably expected to result in placing the individual's health in serious jeopardy, serious impairment to bodily functions, or serious dysfunction of any bodily organ or part." Examples include a pregnant woman in active labor, overdoses, myocardial infarction, and a multitude of other problems.

LEAVING AGAINST MEDICAL ADVICE

A competent patient cannot be held against his or her will. When a patient has been seen by the physician and decides to leave before treatment is complete, the patient is leaving against medical advice (AMA). Risks associated with leaving before treatment is complete should be carefully explained and evidence of the patient's competence documented. Ask the patient to sign an AMA form that explains risks and confirms the patient's decision to leave. Regardless of why the patient is leaving, make sure that the patient knows that he or she can return at any time. If there are any questions regarding the patient's competence, the physician should evaluate the patient to determine competence. Notify appropriate services if an incompetent patient leaves.

Institutions may use a separate term and release form for patients who leave before they are seen by the physician (e.g., left before being seen, left without being seen, left without seeing the physician). These patients are distinguished from patients who leave AMA, because a physician has not seen the patient.

MANAGED CARE ISSUES

Increased enrollment in managed care plans such as health maintenance organizations (HMO) and preferred provider organizations (PPO) has changed the business side of health care. Despite requirements for specific physicians and hospitals, the patient should be treated in the same manner as other patients. Triage and the MSE must be done before discussing insurance or finance. Federal EMTALA regulations take priority over insurance companies' expectations. Many facilities discuss financial issues at the end of the visit to avoid potential EMTALA problems. Refusal by an insurance company to pay for care given by out-of-plan physicians or out-of-plan hospitals should never be considered refusal of treatment. Only the patient can refuse treatment. Stable patients may be transferred to another facility as required by their insurance plan after the MSE has been completed and the patient has agreed to the transfer.

Key Concept
The EMTALA requirement for a medical screening examination has priority over insurance company directives to send the patient to a hospital in his or her network.

AMERICANS WITH DISABILITIES ACT

The Americans With Disabilities Act (ADA) of 1990 guarantees certain rights to individuals with disabilities. Individuals affected by this legislation include those who are physically disabled, visually impaired, or hearing impaired. Requirements include handicapped-accessible bathrooms, wheelchair ramps, lower buttons on elevators for patients in wheelchairs, braille signage, and closed-caption televisions.

The triage nurse must ensure that patients who fall under ADA mandates are offered appropriate services. Oversized wheelchairs should be available for individuals who require them. Sign language interpreters must be offered to each patient who is hearing impaired and must be provided to every person—patient, family, visitor, employee—who requests one. Telecommunication devices for the deaf (TDD) are required for patients who are hearing impaired and wish to use the telephone. Pay telephone TDDs should be provided for the public.

REPORTING SITUATIONS

Most states require hospitals to report certain patient situations to law enforcement. These include, but are not limited to, sexual assault, child abuse, gunshot wounds, knife wounds, and animal bites. Some states require reports on elder abuse, domestic violence, and suicide attempts. If state law dictates, these reports are made regardless of the patient's wishes.

LEGAL SPECIMEN AND EVIDENCE COLLECTION

The triage nurse may be the first person to identify evidence of crime. For example, the patient with a stab wound or gunshot wound may appear at the triage area seeking treatment or the victim of sexual assault may arrive without benefit of a police escort. The triage nurse must be sensitive to the patient's needs while preserving essential evidence. Without attention to details, valuable evidence may be lost and the case dismissed.

In addition to preserving evidence, the triage nurse may be required to collect certain legal specimens. Individuals charged with driving under the influence may be asked to provide blood and urine. Blood, urine, saliva, and semen may be obtained from those charged with rape. Evidence kits with instructions for sexual assault cases and kits for collecting blood and urine for legal analysis are available. Evidence collection must follow specific guidelines to ensure integrity of the evidence and preserve the chain of custody.

ADVANCE DIRECTIVES

The Patient Self-Determination Act (1991) provides patients with a formal mechanism for establishing their beliefs and desires regarding life support measures. The patient can complete an advance directive or living will document that explains the patient's wishes and identifies an individual responsible for making decisions about health care if the patient is unable to do so. Each patient admitted to the hospital should be asked about advance directives (JCAHO, 1998). A copy of the document is placed in the medical record. The triage nurse may ask patients about advance directives in your institution; however, this is not the normal practice for most EDs.

PATIENT RESTRAINTS

Patient injury and even death have occurred with use of restraints (JCAHO, 1998). JCAHO has implemented stringent requirements for applying restraints and monitoring patients in restraints in an effort to decrease use of restraints and to protect patients. Today's violent society makes it unlikely that restraints will ever be eliminated from the ED; however, use of alternatives may decrease use of restraints. Chapter 7: Violence reviews these procedures in greater detail.

SUMMARY

Variability with regard to legal issues from state to state and institution to institution affects the triage nurse. Become familiar with laws in the state where you work and the policies in your institution. Placing the patient's best interest first and adhering strictly to these guidelines is the best protection for you and your patients.

References

Emergency Nurses Association. (1997). <u>Triage: Meeting the challenge</u>. Park Ridge, IL: Author.

Health Care Financing Administration (HCFA). (1998). <u>Revised interpretative guidelines: State operations manual provider certification</u> Washington, DC: Department of Health and Human Services, Health Care Financing Administration. [Transmittal No. 2].

Joint Commission on Accreditation of Healthcare Organizations (JCAHO). (1998). <u>Comprehensive accreditation manual for hospital: The official handbook</u>. Chicago: Author.

Jordan, K. (Ed.). (2000). <u>Emergency nursing core curriculum</u> (5th ed.). Philadelphia: Saunders.

Kitt, S., Selfridge-Thomas, J., Proehl, J., & Kaiser, J. (1995). <u>Emergency nursing: A physiologic and clinical perspective</u> (2nd ed.). Philadelphia: Saunders.

Mitchell, P. (1999). Latest study on telephone triage raises doubts on widespread use. <u>Lancet, 353</u>(9160), 1247.

Newberry, L. (Ed.). (1998). <u>Sheehy's emergency nursing: Principles and practice</u> (4th ed.). St. Louis: Mosby.

1. The key legal element that must be documented in the medical record by the triage nurse is:
   a. Medical history and medication allergies
   b. History of symptoms associated with chief complaint
   c. Mode of arrival at the facility
   d. Presenting complaint and description of patient's status

2. Treatment in the ED against the patient's "will" is acceptable when:
   a. A family member gives permission for treatment
   b. The patient exhibits irrational behavior
   c. The patient is intoxicated or under the influence of drugs
   d. There is a danger of significant morbidity or loss of life

3. The Emergency Medical Treatment and Active Labor Act (EMTALA) requires that a patient presenting to the ED must:
   a. Provide written consent for treatment
   b. Receive a medical screening examination
   c. Be seen by a physician
   d. Contact his or her managed care provider

4. Written consent for treatment is not required if the patient:
   a. Is an emancipated minor
   b. Is physically unable to sign the chart
   c. Does not speak English as a primary language
   d. Has alcohol on the breath

5. The most prudent approach to telephone triage is to:
   a. Encourage the caller seeking advice to seek emergency care
   b. Give minimal advice based on principles of first aid
   c. Deviate from ED protocols when there is a clear need to individualize the advice
   d. Get the patient's telephone number and then call the patient back before you give any advice

6. A patient with a sprained ankle and strong pedal pulses can be sent to his or her private orthopedist's office if:

a. The insurance provider approves this care before the patient leaves the ED

b. The patient refuses the medical screening exam

c. The physician is in the office waiting on the patient

d. X-rays are done before the patient leaves

The purpose of these exercises is to provide specific examples for review of your institution's policies and procedures related to:

- consent for treatment
- telephone advice
- AMA
- notification of authority
- release of information
- transfer to another facility

1. A female calls the triage desk and asks if Mrs. Doe has been brought into the ED from a car crash. Can you legally answer her question? What policies and procedures in your ED direct the triage nurse's decisions in this case scenario?

2. An elderly male who appears intoxicated is brought to the ED by friends who think he is acting "funny." The patient is staggering and yelling, "You can't touch me!" He has an obvious laceration on the forehead with minimal bleeding. Can you force this patient to remain in your ED? What policies and procedures in your ED direct the triage nurse's decisions in this situation?

3. A male calls the ED and asks if he should come in for treatment of abdominal pain. What is your response to this patient based ED policies and procedures regarding telephone triage and advice?

4. A female patient states that her husband beat her. She does not want the police to be notified. What is your response to this patient based on ED policies and procedures regarding notification of legal authorities?

5. A pregnant female arrives in the ED stating she is in labor. This is her first pregnancy and her due date is 3 weeks away. The patient insists that she cannot make it to another hospital that is approved by her managed care provider. a) Are you obligated to examine her? b) What policies and procedures in your ED direct the triage nurse's decisions in this case scenario?

Customer Service *chapter 5*

OBJECTIVES

After completing this chapter, you will be able to:

1. Describe three types of customers in the ED.

2. Identify five behaviors associated with effective customer relations.

3. Articulate the primary purpose of customer service in triage.

RESOURCES

- Hospital and department philosophy, mission statement, and code of conduct

- Formal customer service programs, if applicable

- Letters from satisfied and dissatisfied customers

- Fliers and registration forms for customer service classes

INTRODUCTION

The advent of managed care has had a tremendous effect on how health care organizations do business. Corporations contract with hospitals and health systems to provide care for thousands of employees. Quality clinical care and quality customer service are expected. When a health care organization does not meet the customer's expectations, it can lose not just one dissatisfied customer but thousands if an entire contract is lost. In today's competitive health care market, lost contracts mean lost jobs. Consider customer service skills in the same light as clinical skills. Your job is in jeopardy if you do not have both.

> **Key Concept**
> **Customer service is just as important as clinical skill to the triage nurse and the organization.**

A customer is a "person with whom one must deal" ("Webster's II New Riverside University Dictionary," 1984). The customer may be within your organization or company or he or she may originate from the outside. External customers are individuals who originate from outside the work area. Patients, family, and visitors are external customers. Insurance companies, and ambulance, fire, and police personnel are also external customers. Internal customers are based in the organization or the work area. These are individuals essential to work completion. Registration clerks, nurses in other areas of the hospital, radiology staff, lab personnel, and physicians are the ED's internal customers.

BASIC SKILLS

Customer service is an inherent part of patient care and human interactions. Politeness, courtesy, and respect are just as important for the triage nurse as for the cashier at the grocery store or receptionist at the gas company. The triage nurse encounters more individuals in crisis; however, other aspects of these three jobs are similar. All three individuals deal with the public and may face angry, hostile, or intoxicated customers. These individuals are also the frontline for their organizations. A poor impression during this first crucial encounter can affect how the customer perceives the entire organization. The golden rule for customer service is to treat others as you would like to be treated. The ability to do this involves verbal skill, body language, and acceptance of the customer. Table 5-1 highlights basic customer service skills.

> **Key Concept**
> **Treat each and every patient as you wish to be treated.**

Table 5-1. Basics of Customer Service

- Treat the person with respect.
- Be polite.
- Listen. Give the person your full attention.
- Speak slowly and clearly. Do not speak loudly unless you identify that the person has a hearing problem.
- Apologize if you are interrupted.
- Ask questions to clarify understanding. Paraphrase the complaint to confirm understanding.
- Be sensitive to nonverbal cues.
- Maintain privacy and confidentiality.

Chaos in the triage area and the ED does not mean customer service should suffer. High volume and high acuity are no excuse for rudeness. How then do you keep customer service and clinical skill on the same plane? Building a foundation of effective customer service skills and practicing these skills routinely make it easier to maintain these skills during times of stress and tension. As you develop your own customer service technique, remember the following rules for customer relations. The customer:

- Is the most important person in any business.

- Is not dependent on you—you are dependent on the customer.

- Is not an interruption of your work—he or she is the purpose for it.

- Does you a favor when he or she calls—you are not doing the customer a favor by serving him or her.

- Is a part of your business—not an outsider.

- Is not a cold statistic—he or she is a flesh-and-blood human being with feelings and emotions like your own.

- Is someone who brings you his or her wants—it is your job to fill those wants.

- Deserves the most courteous and attentive treatment you can give him or her.
- Is the life blood of this and every business (Gerson, 1992).

CUSTOMERS

Today's society is not conditioned for waiting. Fast food, take-out service, fast copy services, drive-through banking, and short checkout lines at the grocery store were all developed to meet the desire for instant service. These same services have decreased the public's tolerance for waiting regardless of the reason. Long wait times in the ED are even more frustrating for the patient who is ill or injured. Waiting increases anxiety and can lead to frank hostility in some situations. Lack of information about the wait only worsens the situation. The triage nurse should provide as much information as possible to make the wait more tolerable. Be truthful. Don't promise that the wait is only a "few minutes" if you know it is already 2 hours. It is better to overestimate than underestimate wait time.

In an ideal world, patients understand that those with more serious problems come first. Realistically, this may not be the case. To the patient, his or her problem is an emergency and requires immediate attention. The patient with a laceration may not understand why he is waiting while staff care for victims of a car crash. Accept this, apologize for the wait, and assure the patient that he or she will be seen as soon as possible.

Key Concept
Overestimate how long the patient will wait.

Patients are also exposed to unusual sights, sounds, and smells during the wait. Be sensitive to interactions in the waiting area. Intervene when possible by moving certain individuals to other waiting areas. Place patients with offensive odors or soiled clothing in separate waiting areas whenever possible. Moving intoxicated patients out of the main waiting area is also helpful.

Establishing rapport with the patient as he or she enters can make it easier to interact during the wait. Acknowledge the patient and the problem during the first conversation. Present a welcoming, helpful demeanor. Greet the patient by his or her appropriate title and name. If you do not know the patient's name, use Sir or Ma'am. Do not call patients by their first name unless asked to do so. Remember the importance of body language. Establish eye contact and welcome the patient with a smile. If you are sitting behind a desk, lean forward in a welcoming manner or stand to greet the patient. If you are standing, step toward the patient. Do not cross your arms or put your hands on your hips. These positions convey an attitude of judgment or confrontation and do not offer a sense of welcome. Chewing gum or blowing bubbles is inappropriate at any time. Touching the patient to assess skin temperature and moisture is indicated for most patients, but it should be done in the right context. Establish rapport first, and then touch the patient's hand.

As you interact with patients who are waiting, offer information in a positive way. Negative comments make the situation worse. Telling the patient the wait is because of a slow doctor does not serve you, the facility, or the doctor. Blaming other departments (e.g., lab, x-ray, ICU) is also inappropriate. These comments do not make patients feel secure about the care they are receiving. Offer comments in a positive context. "The department is full so there is a wait. I am right here if you have any questions. Please let me know if there is anything I can do while you wait." Other ways to make the wait more tolerable include providing magazines and television. Keep the television set on a channel with broad appeal.

CONFLICT RESOLUTION

Violence is a real threat for the triage nurse. Do not place yourself or your patients at risk. Be sensitive to situations that lead to conflict and gracefully resolve problems as they arise. If a patient becomes angry and verbally attacks you, do not take it personally. Speak in a normal volume and tone. Shouting at the patient makes the situation worse. Do not defend yourself or the institution. Focus on the customer's feelings and concerns. Logic takes second place to emotions in these situations. Do what you can within the limits of your job as the triage nurse. If you cannot resolve the situation, you should then involve the charge nurse or department manager. Summon help if the patient becomes violent. Do not attempt to subdue the patient without assistance. Chapter 7: Violence discusses recognition and management of the violent patient.

SUMMARY

Customer service skills are essential for the triage nurse. Patients who leave the waiting room dissatisfied tell their family, their neighbors, and their coworkers. In today's competitive health care market, this type of bad press affects the bottom line. By using effective customer service skills, the triage nurse can make a difference to the patient by decreasing anxiety and to the organization by positively affecting the patient's perception of the organization.

References

Gerson, R.F. (1992). <u>Beyond customer service: Keeping customers happy for life</u>. Menlo Park, CA: Crisp Publications.

<u>Webster's II New Riverside University Dictionary</u>. (1984). Boston: Riverside Publishing.

1. The most appropriate greeting when a patient approaches the triage desk is "Hello, my name is__________," and then
   a. What is your problem today?
   b. How can I help you?
   c. Write your name and date of birth on this sheet.
   d. Who is your doctor?

2. The primary cause of conflict in the triage area is:
   a. Lack of a private physician
   b. Unmet expectations
   c. Cost of emergency services
   d. Wait times

3. Identify five actions or behaviors that can be included in your initial triage conversation that will help establish good customer relations.

   -
   -
   -
   -
   -

4. Define three types of ED customers and explain why it is important to establish positive customer relations with them.

   -
   -
   -

5. Describe essential steps in resolving conflict.

6. Define the purpose of customer service for the triage area.

7. Describe the best course of action when a patient becomes angry and is attempting to leave without seeing the physician.

1. Describe how customer service is addressed in the triage area at your facility.

2. Review resources for customer service problems in the triage area.

3. Discuss management of a verbally abusive customer in the triage area.

Cultural and Religious Considerations

chapter 6

OBJECTIVES

After completing this chapter, you will be able to:

1. Explain the significance of understanding cultural diversity in triage.

2. Describe techniques for gaining information about the patient's culture and health belief practices.

3. Discuss two problems associated with using an interpreter and identify two interventions to minimize the language barrier.

RESOURCES

- Cultural references
- Language references
- Lists of interpreters
- Policies related to interpreters and language lines

INTRODUCTION

No matter where you live and work, you are more likely today than ever before to encounter individuals who do not share your cultural origins and beliefs. This is particularly true in the ED. Understanding and accepting another person's cultural beliefs are essential for providing care in the ED. The ability to ascertain essential information about the patient in triage requires sensitivity to the person's culture. Culture does not refer to where a person lives, the color of his or her skin, or where his or her grandparents were born. Leininger (1985) defined culture as "values, beliefs, norms, and practices of a particular group that are learned and shared and that guide thinking, decisions, and actions in a patterned way (p. 209)." An individual's culture is characterized by variations in communication, time, space, biology, social organization, and environment (Newberry, 1998).

The Joint Commission on Accreditation of Healthcare Organizations (JCAHO) (1998) requires assessment of cultural, religious, and spiritual needs for every patient. The purpose of this assessment is to identify specific needs in these areas and to use this information to plan the patient's care. Recognition of primary cultural groups seen in the ED can facilitate this assessment. Prior study of cultural practices for the dominant groups makes it easier to assess cultural needs.

CULTURAL PRACTICES

Cultural practices play a significant role in perception of health care and the health care provider. One cultural group may see the "good nurse" as the one that hovers over the patient or is constantly in attendance, whereas another cultural group may view this as invasive behavior (Leininger, 1985). Comprehensive discussion of specific cultural practices for various groups is beyond the scope of this text; however, a brief discussion is provided. Table 6-1 outlines select cultural beliefs related to health care. You are encouraged to expand your study of these and other cultural groups encountered in your practice area.

Table 6-1. Cultural Beliefs Regarding Health Care

Cultural Group	Belief	Common Health Problems
African-American	•Using the patient's first name without permission is considered disrespectful. •Considerable variations exist in health attitudes and behaviors. •The family is oriented around women. •Illness occurs because of disharmony in life. •Some may believe in folk medicine, voodoo, witchcraft, and magic.	•Hypertension, coronary artery disease, diabetes mellitus, sickle cell anemia
Appalachian	•Illness is the will of God. •Folk medicine is very important. •Eye contact is considered very rude. •The focus is on the state of the blood—thick or thin, high or low, good or bad. •There is an inherent distrust of hospitals.	•Tuberculosis, diabetes mellitus, coronary artery disease
Arabic	•Disease is caused by evil eye. •Illness and/or injury are the will of God. •Little information about self or family is given to strangers. •Health caregivers are seen as personal employees. •Any display of flesh is considered pornographic.	•Urinary infections, cardiovascular disease, diabetes mellitus, thalassemia
Cambodian	•Imbalance causes "wind illness." Coin rubbing, cupping, or other dermal abrasive techniques are used to release the bad winds. •Only close relatives should touch the head. •Pain may be severe before relief is requested.	•Chloroquine resistant malaria
Chinese	•Physical contact with strangers is uncomfortable. •Accepting something when first offered is rude. •Hospitals are a place to die. •Illness is an imbalance between yin and yang. •Do not accept pain medicine when first offered.	•Hypertension, liver cancer, stomach cancer, lactose intolerance, diabetes
Cuban	•Hand gestures are important for communication. •Illness is caused by supernatural powers such as evil eye. Magic spells are the only treatment. •Verbal expression of pain acceptable.	•Diabetes mellitus, lactose intolerance
Eastern Indian	•Illness is an imbalance between body, fire, earth, wind, space, and water. •Quiet acceptance of pain.	•Anemia in women, vitamin A deficiency

Table 6-1. Cultural Beliefs Regarding Health Care cont.

Cultural Group	Belief	Common Health Problems
Egypt	•Health dictated by Allah, so often take a passive role in health care. •Evil eye and hot/cold disease factors co-exist with Western medical practices. •Injections perceived as more effective than pills and liquids. •Amulets with sacred verses or stones may be worn. •Expect immediate pain relief.	•Chloroquine-sensitive malaria is endemic.
Ethiopia	•Magico-religious. •Amulets may be worn for protection against disease. •May use bloodletting to treat malaria. •May refuse pain medications.	•Yellow fever, chloroquine-resistant malaria. AIDS.
Greece	•Bio-medical, magico-religious. •Protective beads or stone charms may be worn. •Passive reactions to pain are practiced.	•β-Thalassemia, Mediterranean-type G6PD deficiency, familial Mediterranean fever.
Japanese	•Illness is an imbalance between the person and the universe. •Isoniazid may be inactive in Japanese patients. •The effects of succinylcholine are prolonged.	•Hypertension, liver cancer, stomach cancer, lactose intolerance
Laotian	•Illness is caused by bad winds. Winds are released by scratching or pinching until red lines or marks appear. •There is a strong belief in herbal medicine. •Parents are the only ones allowed to touch the top of a child's head. •Pain must be severe before relief is requested.	•Tuberculosis •Iodine deficiency
Mexican-American	•Health is harmony between the social and spiritual world. Disease occurs because of an imbalance between hot and cold. •There is a strong belief in evil eye and hexes. •A child's head may be shaved to treat a respiratory illness.	•Diabetes mellitus, lactose intolerance, tuberculosis
Native American	•Each tribe or nation has its own language, religion, and beliefs. •Health is a balance between the social and spiritual world. •Children are very independent. Parents may not be aware of a child's recent behaviors. •Patients may metabolize ethanol differently.	•Lactose intolerance, alcoholism, cirrhosis, diabetes mellitus, heart disease
Vietnamese	•Illness is caused by bad winds. Skin is rubbed with coins or other abrasives to release winds. •Touching the top of a child's head is not acceptable.	•Tuberculosis, hepatitis, cholera, typhoid

(Geissler, 1998)

LANGUAGE BARRIERS

Language is often the first and most obvious source of cultural conflict between the triage nurse and the patient (ENA, 1997). The triage nurse may recognize obvious problems such as broken bones or lacerations without the benefit of words; however, verbal communication is essential to fully assess the patient and determine important historical information. Many EDs have full-time interpreters available, whereas others use on-call interpreters. Language lines (e.g., AT&T) provide access to more than 100 language interpreters, but cost may be a concern. Using family members as interpreters is not without problems.

The ability to speak a given language does not necessarily include a familiarity with jargon and professional terms. Ideally, the interpreter is familiar with these and other aspects of the languages of both the triage nurse and the patient. The interpreter needs to translate information from the triage nurse's educational or intellectual level to the patient's level. Jargon and professional terms must be decoded and expressed in terms the patient can understand. This decoding and translation may be difficult if words do not have the same context when translated. This is true even for English words. For example, a word that means dance or dancing in one country may be an obscenity in another.

Social level, personal characteristics, gender, and other unrecognized factors may skew communication despite the interpreter's level of expertise. There are no easy answers to this challenge. The best action for the triage nurse is to utilize all available resources and remain sensitive to cultural variations within the area.

RELIGIOUS PRACTICES

Religious beliefs may be determined by culture; however, this is not always the case. Table 6-2 briefly outlines various religious groups and their beliefs. Again, this should not be viewed as a comprehensive guide. If you are not sure of the person's beliefs, ask the patient.

Table 6-2. Religious Considerations

Religion	Health Practices
Baptist	•Some believe in "laying on of hands."
Black Muslim	•Alcohol and pork are prohibited. •Faith healing is not acceptable.
Buddhist	•Some sects are strict vegetarians. •Alcohol and drug use is discouraged. •The body should be left as it is at death and covered with a sheet. No one should touch the hand or close the mouth and eyes.
Catholic	•No meat is consumed on Friday. •Contraception and abortion are unacceptable. •Religious articles are important. •Amputated body parts should be buried. •The Sacrament of Anointing of the Sick is given to those with serious illness and at time of death.
Christian Scientist	•Medications or blood transfusions are not accepted. •Immunizations are limited to those required by law.

Table 6-2. Religious Considerations cont.

Religion	Health Practices
Church of God	•Members observe beliefs surrounding clean and unclean meat as described in the Bible.
Church of Jesus Christ of Latter-Day Saints	•Members do not smoke, or drink alcohol, tea, or coffee. They eat meat sparingly. •Members believe in anointments or laying on of hands. •Members may wear special garments.
Eastern Orthodox	•Restrictions depend on the specific sect.
Episcopal	•Some believe in faith healing. •Religious icons are very important.
Greek Orthodox	•A health crisis is handled by an ordained priest. •Autopsies are discouraged.
Hare Krishna	•Members do not eat meat, fish, or eggs and do not drink alcohol.
Hinduism	•Believers eat no beef, pork, or veal and may be strict vegetarians. •Believers prefer to die at home. •Autopsies are not encouraged.
Islam	•Members do not eat pork or pork byproducts. •Members do not drink or take any intoxicants. •After death, the patient's arms and legs should be straightened, eyes should be closed, and mouth shut with a bandage.
Jehovah's Witness	•Blood transfusions are not allowed. •Members will eat nothing to which blood has been added. •Organ donation is not supported.
Judaism	•There are numerous dietary kosher laws. Believers usually do not eat pork. •Amputated body parts must be buried. •Burial must take place within 24 hours of death. The body is attended until burial.
Lutheran	•Anointments are important.
Methodist	•Communion is important. •Donation of body parts is encouraged.
Pentecostal	•Some abstain from alcohol and do not eat pork.
Orthodox Presbyterian	•Pastor or elder is called for ill person.
Russian Orthodox	•Members believe in divine healing. •The cross necklace is very important. •Autopsy, embalming, or cremation is discouraged.
Salvation Army	•Members abstain from alcohol, tobacco, and nonprescription drugs.
Seventh Day Adventist	•Members abstain from alcohol, tobacco, and drugs found in cola, tea, and coffee.
Unitarian Universalist	•Members believe that God helps those who help themselves. •Some clergy do not make hospital visits.

(Miller, 1995; Newberry, 1998; Ontario Multifaith Council on Spiritual and Religious Care, 1995; Wong, 1993;)

SUMMARY

The triage nurse is often the first person encountered by individuals seeking health care. Sensitivity to the beliefs of each person is essential if the patient's needs are to be identified and resolved. Understanding and accepting the unique characteristics of the person's culture help establish rapport and facilitate communication. Identification of language barriers and resolution of the barrier through use of appropriate interpreters is also necessary.

References

Geissler, E.M. (1998). <u>Pocket guide to cultural assessment</u> (2nd ed.). St. Louis: Mosby.

Joint Commission on Accreditation of Healthcare Organizations (JCAHO). (1998). <u>Comprehensive accreditation manual for hospitals: The official handbook</u>. Chicago: Author.

Leininger, M. (1985). Transcultural care, diversity and universality: A theory of nursing. <u>Nursing Health Care, 6</u>(4), 209.

Miller, J. (1995). Caring for Cambodian refugees in the ED. <u>Journal of Emergency Nursing, 21</u>(6), 498-502.

Newberry, L. (Ed.). (1998). <u>Sheehy's emergency nursing: Principles and practice</u> (4th ed.). St. Louis: Mosby.

Ontario Multifaith Council on Spiritual and Religious Care. (1995). <u>Multifaith information manual</u>. Toronto, On: Author.

Wong, D. (1993). <u>Whaley & Wong's essentials of pediatric nursing</u> (4th ed.). St. Louis: Mosby.

1. Factors that contribute to language barriers in the triage setting include use of jargon and professional terms. Select the most appropriate statement for the patient with a language barrier.
   a. Who is your primary care provider?
   b. What brought you to the ED?
   c. Where on your body do you hurt?
   d. Do you have any known medication allergies?

2. The Joint Commission on Accreditation of Healthcare Organizations (JCAHO) requires the ED nurse to assess all adult patients for:
   a. Height
   b. Spiritual needs
   c. Primary care provider
   d. Managed care provider

3. Individual culture is characterized by variations in which of the following?
   a. Race
   b. Gender
   c. Communication
   d. Geography

4. Examples of problems related to cultural misunderstanding include:
   a. Assessment of hypertension in African-American patients
   b. Keeping all skin except the hands and eyes covered for Middle Eastern females
   c. Reporting a Cambodian father for child abuse when you observe him rubbing coins on his child's chest and back
   d. Limiting physical contact with a Chinese patient

5. Cultural and religious beliefs—regardless of group or affiliation—affect which of the following?
   a. Sexual orientation
   b. Skin color
   c. Chosen profession
   d. Dietary regimen

1. List resources available in your ED that address cultural diversity.

2. Discuss the procedure for obtaining interpreters for major non-English speaking groups as well as other groups. Identify any variations for time of day.

3. Review the procedure for contacting spiritual counselors in your facility. Identify the location of any resource texts and telephone contacts.

OBJECTIVES

After completing this chapter, you will be able to:

1. Identify two patient populations at high-risk for violent behavior.

2. Describe three behaviors used to predict violence.

3. Discuss two approaches to prevent violent behavior.

RESOURCES

- Policies related to restraint and seclusion

- Procedures to call security and law enforcement

- Lockdown procedures and other security measures

INTRODUCTION

Violence is a reality in the world at large and in the hospital. Homicide is the second leading cause of all work-related deaths in this country, and it is the leading cause of work-related deaths in women (US Department of Labor, 1996). Williams and Robertson (1997) described two general forms of violence that frequently occur in hospitals. Physical violence is any physical act that causes injury to another person or property. Acts of aggression are verbal or physical actions used to cause fear.

Health care workers are 16 times more likely to be injured in the workplace than other types of workers (Elliott, 1997). Unique features that make hospital personnel vulnerable to attack are described in Table 7-1.

The reality is that staff in the ED are at greater risk for violence than other hospital employees. Fifty percent of all hospital assaults are reported in the ED (Stultz, 1994). More than 90% of emergency nurses have reported verbal abuse, and 87% have reported physical abuse (ENA, 1994). With increasing violence in schools, the workplace, and other previously "safe" areas, it is imperative that emergency nurses remain alert to the potential for violence and intervene appropriately.

> **Key Concept**
> **The threat of violence is a reality for the emergency nurse. Protect yourself and your patients by remaining alert to the potential for violence.**

The ENA position statement "Violence in the Emergency Setting" notes six primary factors leading to ED violence (ENA, 1991). Long waits, staff shortages, ED overcrowding, availability of drugs and potential hostages, easy access, and presence of patients with alcohol and drug problems were factors 10 years ago and are just as critical today. The magnitude of these issues has increased significantly in the past decade. Lack of a pre-existing relationship with the patient as well as the inherent chaos and stress of the ED increases the potential for violence.

Table 7-1. Factors That Increase the Risk for Violence In Hospitals

Origin	Factor	Description
Patients, families, visitors	Unrestricted setting	•A 24-hour open door policy allows individuals easy access and movement from one place to another within the hospital (Elliott, 1997).
	Patient population	•Patients may abuse drugs or alcohol, may be gang members, or may have a history of violence or mental illness.
	Inability to cope	•Trauma or a sudden, catastrophic illness may increase stress beyond the patient or family's ability to cope.
	Societal changes	•There is easy access to drugs, alcohol, and guns. •Patients with acute and chronic mental health conditions can refuse medication or treatment in certain circumstances.
	Robbery	•Drugs and money available in the hospital are prime targets for desperate thieves (Williams & Robertson, 1997).
	Illness and drugs	•Systemic disorders, toxic levels of certain drugs, and various neurologic disorders can result in violent behavior.
	Revenge	•An individual who feels there has been a lack of attention or improper treatment can become violent, particularly in the ED. (Simonowitz, 1996).
Fellow employees	Downsizing	•Disgruntled employees may become violent (Williams & Robertson, 1997).
	Unhappy employees	•Those who feel no control over the environment or job assignment may become violent (Williams & Robertson, 1997).

The advent of technology to monitor turnaround times and identify bottlenecks has done little to decrease ED wait times. Other factors such as an increasing volume of patients, staff shortages in supporting departments (e.g., lab, x-ray) and increasing patient acuity have made the wait even longer. This can lead to havoc in the waiting area and presents a challenge for the triage nurse. Patients and families are already under stress because of the problem that brought them to the ED. A long wait in a crowded, noisy waiting room just increases the stress. Appropriate and timely interventions by the triage nurse can defuse a violent response and prevent catastrophe.

HIGH-RISK PATIENT POPULATIONS

Violent behavior is associated with low tolerance for frustration, problems with authority, limited resources, and poor coping skills. Many patients who come to the ED have a significant potential for violence. Patients with psychiatric or organic disorders resulting in acute confusion are two populations most likely to behave violently.

The most common psychiatric diagnoses related to violent behavior are bipolar disorder (manic phase with psychotic symptoms) and paranoid schizophrenia. A patient with delusions, particularly paranoid delusions, is also at risk. The patient may believe that violence is justified as a defense against those he or she believes are plotting against him or her.

Organic causes of violent behavior include head injury, hypoglycemia, hypoxia, postic-
tal state, dementia, and—the most common cause of violent behavior—alcohol or drug
toxicity and withdrawal. Any organic disorder that alters metabolic or neurologic equi-
librium and impedes the ability to think logically can lead to violence. Confusion and
poor impulse control found in patients with dementia and organic brain disorders
increase the risk for violence. Alcohol intoxication is associated with uninhibited
behavior, increased emotional liability, and impaired judgment. Cocaine, amphetamines, and other stimulants are associated with increased irritability, psychomotor
agitation, and suspicion. Stimulants are also noted for causing "superhuman strength",
which makes the violence even more destructive.

PREDICTORS OF VIOLENT BEHAVIOR

Violence does not happen in isolation; it occurs in incremental phases. Two phases
of previolent behavior precede the violent outburst. Previolent phase I is characterized by subtle verbal and nonverbal clues to violence. Verbal interventions are
usually effective during this phase (Drury, 1999). Violence is imminent during
previolent phase II. Individuals in this phase do not generally respond to verbal
interventions. Table 7-2 summarizes indicators for violent behavior.

As the triage nurse, you must remain alert. Do not ignore your gut instinct or inner
voices. If you feel uncomfortable or frightened during the interview, you may be
responding to subtle clues from the patient. Some patients may purposefully try to
provoke defensive statements by insulting you or making obnoxious statements.

Key Concept
Do not ignore your gut instinct. If you feel unsafe,
stop the interview and get help.

Table 7-2. Indicators of Impending Violence	
Patient	**Characteristic**
Appearance	•Piercing stare
	•Narrow, glaring eyes
	•Red face—veins may be "popping out"
	•Fearful or angry expression
	•Perspiring heavily
Demeanor	•Talking rapidly
	•Repeating the same thing over and over
	•Chanting or singing
	•Interacting in a euphoric or grandiose manner indicative of a manic state
	•Making delusional, paranoid statements
	•Admitting to hearing voices
	•Using a loud, angry, screaming voice

Table 7-2. Indicators of Impending Violence cont.

Patient	Characteristic
Demeanor cont.	•Using profanity •Making aggressive or threatening statements •Pacing, fidgeting, unable to sit still •Clenching and unclenching hands •Pounding fists •Making exaggerated movements •Tensing muscles •Frequently changing position •Rocking upper body while sitting •Carrying a weapon (Drury, 1999, POV, 1998; Williams & Robertson, 1997)
Behavior	•Hostile, threatening, belligerent, confused, suspicious, throwing things, hitting, pushing, kicking •Soiled clothes, disheveled appearance •Bizarre behavior (Williams & Robertson, 1997)

PATIENT INTERACTIONS

When you identify patients at risk for violence, you must exercise caution to safeguard yourself and other patients. Approach the patient and introduce yourself from a distance. Remain calm and speak in a self-assured voice. Agitated patients may react strongly to fear in health care providers. Interview the patient in an open area when possible. Or, keep the door open and position yourself between the patient and the door. Notify colleagues so they can keep an eye on the situation. Ask the patient "How can I help you?" Do not use medical jargon while speaking to the patient. Intoxicated or verbally abusive patients often respond better to a very low voice, even a whisper in some cases.

> **Key Concept**
> **Never let the patient get between you and the door.**

Maintain a nonthreatening posture. Hold your arms at your side rather than crossing them in front. Avoid a square-on stance. Maintain distance of at least an arm's length so you do not invade the patient's personal space. This position requires the patient to step toward you to attack. Stop the interview and get help if you ever feel unsafe.

Violent episodes occur when the patient feels provoked or threatened. Avoid startling or scaring the patient. Use a low tone of voice and a neutral expression—cheerfulness or excessive concern may be misinterpreted. Violence can be associated with care activities that violate the patient's personal space. Exercise extreme caution when assessment involves removing clothing or when checking pockets or other belongings for identification. Do not touch the patient who appears to be sleeping, distracted, confused, or listening to voices. Avoid reaching or leaning over the patient. Calmly call the patient's name to get his or her attention.

Anxious Patients

Extreme anxiety can progress to agitation or even frank violence in certain situations. When you identify a patient with severe anxiety, listen carefully to what the patient is saying. Ask questions in a simple, direct manner. Encourage the patient to express his or her concerns. Provide support and understanding. If the patient becomes agitated, use a more direct approach.

Agitated Patients

When dealing with an agitated person, avoid actions that may increase frustration or confusion. Do not criticize or make unnecessary requests. Reassure the patient that you are here to help. Acknowledge the person's emotions without being judgmental. Place the person in a less stimulating environment and establish simple, realistic limits on his or her behavior. Build esteem and confidence by recognizing how much strength it takes to remain calm and cooperative; however, do not negotiate on the patient's terms. For example, do not bargain when the patient offers to shut up in return for a cigarette. Do not argue with the patient or defend yourself against accusations. Use a more direct approach when anxiety and fear escalate to hostility and aggression.

PATIENT MANAGEMENT

When anxiety or agitation escalate to violence, the goal is to safeguard the patient and the staff. A team approach is required for patient restraint. Never attempt to subdue the patient alone. Use security, police, or other able-bodied personnel. A show of force may be all it takes, because it tells the patient that his violence is being taken seriously. When a show of force and other alternatives to restraint fail, the patient must be physically restrained to prevent injury to everyone concerned. Restraints may be applied without an order in an emergent situation, but a physician's order must be obtained, eventually usually within one hour (JCAHO, 1998). Restraint orders must be time limited; as-needed restraint orders are not acceptable. The reason for the restraint and failed interventions must be documented.

The violent patient should be restrained on a stretcher with the minimum amount of restraint required to safeguard the patient and others. Usually four or five individuals are required for this procedure. One person controls the patient's head while other team members secure the limbs (Glasson, 1993). Staff should use care to avoid being bitten or spit on during the restraint procedure. Hold the upper extremities at the wrist and shoulder and secure the lower extremities above the knee and at the ankle. Leather restraints or other safety devices may be used to limit movement. After restraints have been applied, the patient should be carefully searched to remove potential weapons. Exercise great caution during the search process, because needles or other sharp objects may be in the patient's pockets.

Violence in the triage area or waiting area is a threat to not only the triage nurse but other patients, family members, and visitors. These individuals should be guided to a safe place to make sure they are not hurt or that they do not become part of the violence. Backup personnel may be required if the violence involves guns or several people. Brawls have occurred in ED waiting rooms.

Weapons

More and more patients come to the hospital with weapons such as knives and guns (Drury, 1999). Some EDs have installed metal detectors at all entrances to identify individuals with weapons so that weapons can be removed before they can be used. Shootings and stabbings in hospitals and EDs have been reported across the country (Elliott, 1997; Fiesta, 1996; Hoag-Apel, 1998, 1999; Point of View [POV], 1998). When you suspect a patient has a gun or other weapon, notify security or designated personnel immediately. Do not confront the individual. Never argue with or attempt to take weapons from a threatening individual. Security and law enforcement are trained to manage these situations. Remove individuals at risk immediately. Your first priority in this situation is to protect yourself and others in the area.

SUMMARY

Pay attention to the world around you. Remember that violence is a very real threat for the triage nurse. You cannot prevent all violent acts, but you can defuse or minimize many potentially violent situations (POV, 1998). Recognizing potentially violent patients and intervening early are the most effective ways to make the ED safer for you and your patients.

References

Drury, T. (1999). How to defuse a walking time bomb. <u>Nursing Management, 30</u>(3), 59-61.

Emergency Nurses Association. (1994). <u>Violence in the emergency setting</u>. Park Ridge, IL: Author.

Emergency Nurses Association. (1994). <u>ENA survey on prevalence of violence in US emergency departments, Appendix B</u>. Park Ridge, IL: Author.

Elliott, P. (1997). Violence in health care: What nurse managers need to know. <u>Nursing Management, 28</u>(12), 38-41.

Glasson, L. (1993). Preparation, staff awareness, preventive practices, and the psychiatric patient. <u>Journal of Emergency Nursing, 19</u>(5), 385-391.

Fiesta, J. (1996). Corporate liability: Security and violence, part I. <u>Nursing Management, 27</u>(3), 14-16.

Hoag-Apel, C. (1998). Violence in the ED. <u>Nursing Management, 29</u>(7), 60-63.

Hoag-Apel, C. (1999). Smart safeguards for the ED: Preventing rising ED violence from striking your unit. <u>Nursing Management, 30</u>(5), 31-33.

Joint Commission on Accreditation of Healthcare Organizations (JCAHO). (1998). <u>Comprehensive accreditation manual for hospitals: The official handbook</u>. Chicago, IL: Author.

Point of View (POV). (1998, August). Violence in the workplace. <u>Point of View Magazine</u>, 4-6.

Simonowitz, J. (1996). Health care workers and workplace violence. <u>Occupational Medicine: State of the Art Reviews, 11</u>(2), 277-291.

Stultz, M. (1994). Crime in hospitals 1992: The latest IAHSS survey. <u>Journal of Health Care Protective Management, 10</u>(2), 1-40.

US Department of Labor. (1996). <u>Protecting community workers against violence</u>. OSHA Program Highlight [Fact Sheet No. OSHA 96-53]. Washington, DC: Author.

Williams, M., & Robertson, K. (1997). Workplace violence: Prevalence, prevention, and first-line interventions. <u>Critical Care Nursing Clinics of North America, 9</u>(2), 221-228.

1. The most effective predictor for potential violence is:
   a. Gut instinct on the part of the triage nurse
   b. Excessive psychomotor activity
   c. History of spousal abuse
   d. Disheveled or bizarre appearance

2. Interventions for the patient who is potentially violent include:
   a. Presenting a cheerful and concerned demeanor
   b. Encouraging the patient to ventilate
   c. Using simple, direct communication
   d. Telling the patient you feel his or her pain

3. The patient who is extremely agitated should be approached with:
   a. A low tone and neutral expression
   b. A strong, forceful voice
   c. Loud, simple directions
   d. A soothing touch to the shoulder

4. Patient behaviors that can predict impending violent behavior do not include:
   a. Increased motor activity
   b. Calm demeanor in the face of questions
   c. Presence of a weapon
   d. Bizarre behavior

5. A combative, hostile, homicidal patient would be considered which level of severity based on the ESI model?
   a. Level 1
   b. Level 2

Clinical Application

1. Describe specific measures the triage nurse should take when a patient becomes violent to ensure personal safety as well as the safety of the patients in the waiting room.

2. Outline the procedure for accessing security from triage. Discuss specific situations that should lead you to contact security.

3. Identify specific situations when the patient should be placed in restraints or seclusion.

4. List behaviors that indicate escalation of violence.

OBJECTIVES

After completing this chapter, you will be able to:

1. Describe three things the triage nurse must know to prepare for incoming disaster patients.

2. Identify two parameters used to assign patients to disaster care areas.

3. Contrast the role of the triage nurse in a disaster to daily ED triage.

RESOURCES

- Hospital disaster plan

- ED-specific disaster plan

- Description of nurse's role in disaster triage

- Community disaster plan

- Decontamination policies

INTRODUCTION

A disaster is defined as a natural or manmade situation that produces patients who need services in numbers that extend beyond immediately available resources (ENA, 2000; Kitt, Selfridge-Thomas, Proehl, & Kaiser, 1995; Newberry, 1998). The situation may involve a large total number of patients with only a small number of patients whose needs place a significant demand on resources. Each facility and ED is unique with regard to location and resources. A situation that depletes resources in one facility may not significantly affect another facility. Table 8-1 highlights situations or events that are commonly associated with disasters.

Table 8-1. Examples of Disasters	
Natural	**Manmade**
•Hurricanes	•Bus, train, or plane crashes
•Tornadoes	•Fires
•Floods	•Collapsed buildings
•Earthquakes	•Bombs
•Landslides	•Hazardous material spills

The key to successful disaster management is to provide care for those in greatest need without depleting resources on those with little or no chance of survival. Appropriate triage is crucial to this endeavor. Each facility must have a disaster or emergency preparedness plan in place (JCAHO, 1998). This chapter provides an overview of disaster triage, but it should be supplemented by review of the facility's disaster plan.

DISASTER NOTIFICATION

Notification of a disaster may occur through various routes of communication. Civil defense or the local emergency management agency may notify the facility by telephone, whereas law enforcement, fire personnel, or EMS personnel may contact the facility by telephone or radio. Calls from the media or private citizens may also occur. The person who receives the call should determine specifics about the event including nature of the incident, location, time, probable injuries, and projected number of victims. It is imperative that the estimated arrival time for first victims be identified. The responsibility for activating the hospital's disaster plan varies with each facility. The triage nurse may be in a position to activate the plan; however, it is more likely that he or she will be responsible only for communicating the information to ED staff.

The triage nurse's role varies with disaster plans. He or she may remain in the triage station and continue to triage nondisaster patients. Another nurse may be assigned to the triage team to meet disaster patients as they arrive. Ideally, the facility's plan is flexible enough to ensure that the most experienced triage nurse joins the disaster triage team.

DISASTER CARE AREAS

Managing large numbers of disaster patients is best done in specific treatment areas—the critical treatment area, the noncritical treatment area, and the minor treatment area. Designation of these areas depends on the number of victims, type of injuries, and the specific facility. Treatment areas may be within the ED or scattered throughout the facility. Ambulatory patients should be separated from the area where ambulance patients arrive.

ROUTINE TRIAGE NURSE FUNCTIONS

In addition to the routine expectations of the triage nurse, he or she has assigned duties during a disaster situation. These duties vary by facility and situation, but usually include controlling the crowd, managing telephone calls, and relaying information. Before disaster patients arrive, patients and families already in the ED should be told that a disaster has occurred and the ED is expecting a large number of patients. Nonurgent patients may be directed to other areas of the hospital or other facilities, or may be asked to leave and return later for treatment. This depends entirely on the facility and the magnitude of the disaster. If the ED continues to see nondisaster patients, routine patient registration should be kept separate from disaster patient registration.

Different disasters create different types of crowds. For example, a school bus crash brings in large numbers of parents, relatives, and school employees, whereas events involving teenagers give rise to large numbers of friends. Regardless of who makes up the disaster "crowd", the triage nurse at the regular triage desk plays a pivotal role in crowd control. As soon as separate waiting areas are set up for those associated with the disaster, the triage nurse must control traffic to these areas while juggling other tasks. These waiting areas may also be used for disaster patients who have been seen and discharged.

When the disaster involves hazardous chemical exposure, the triage nurse must be vigilant in keeping contaminated victims out of the waiting area. Most victims are decontaminated at the scene; however, contaminated patients can still arrive at the door of the ED. Security guards may be posted at the door to help screen contaminated patients, but this does not eliminate the need for vigilance on the part of the triage nurse.

Another aspect of crowd control is handling the media. The triage nurse may be the first person to interact with the media. The facility may designate a specific area for media, but some members of the media may attempt to gain access to the ED and the patients. Contact the appropriate media liaison for your facility. Do not release information to the media unless directed to do so by appropriate facility administrators.

If the triage station routinely fields telephone calls from the public, the advent of a disaster will significantly increase the number of calls. Using a volunteer to manage these calls can be effective. There may also be a large number of telephone calls for employees. Procedures for managing these calls are determined by each facility.

TRIAGE TEAM

In addition to designating specific treatment areas for disaster patients, the facility establishes a triage team. The team should consist of an experienced emergency nurse, an emergency physician, and a registration clerk. The team establishes the triage area where patients arrive—on the ambulance ramp, parking lot, or ED entrance. Identification of the team is essential. The most effective techniques are use of hats or vests which are more visible than armbands. If there are large numbers of victims, two triage teams may be needed.

The emergency nurse assesses disaster victims and makes triage decisions. He or she may also designate treatment areas. The emergency physician may assist with triage, perform life-saving procedures such as needle thoracostomy or pronounce fatally wounded patients dead. The registration clerk manages premade charts and bands each patient. The clerk may also maintain a log of patients and their destination. The better the communication between the triage team and the treatment areas, the smoother the system flows. Walkie-talkies or other closed circuit communication devices are ideal. These devices allow the team to alert disaster care areas regarding incoming patients. In turn, coordinators in the care areas can update the triage team of their availability for more patients.

Key Concept
Communication between the triage area and treatment area is essential for smooth patient movement.

TRIAGE OF VICTIMS

The first victims to arrive are often not the most seriously injured. If the disaster was in the immediate area, patients can arrive in private vehicles driven by well-meaning volunteers. These patients should be appropriately triaged so they do not interfere with care of more serious patients who arrive later.

The first patients to arrive by ambulance are the most critically injured if field triage has been appropriately performed. However, it is not unusual for critically injured patients to arrive later as emergency personnel move from the perimeter of the disaster scene to the center. This is particularly true of fires and explosions where victims closest to the center are more seriously injured. Patients who require extrication also arrive later. Table 8-2 gives examples of the conditions of patients who fall within the four triage categories.

Critical Patients

Patients who require immediate care to save their lives should go to the critical treatment area. This area should be located as close to the triage area as possible. Examples of patients requiring immediate care include those with airway compromise, hemorrhage, or those receiving cardiopulmonary resuscitation with a reasonable chance of recovery.

Fatally Injured Patients

Resuscitative measures are not started on patients who have little or no hope of recovery. Patients who have no pulse, are apneic, and have obvious fatal injuries should be triaged to the morgue. Patients with fatal injuries who still have vital signs should be triaged to an area where comfort care can be given until death occurs.

Patients with no vital signs who do not have obvious fatal injuries present the greatest dilemma. These patients can consume valuable resources and supplies while other critically ill but salvageable patients wait for care. These patients may be sent to the critical care area where simple resuscitation measures (e.g., defibrillation, a fluid challenge) are instituted. If there is no response, resuscitative measures can be terminated.

Noncritical Patients

Patients with injuries that do not require immediate attention but could be life-threatening if ignored are sent to the noncritical area. These patients often require admission, surgery, and intravenous analgesia. Patients with long-bone fractures and moderate burns fall into this category.

Patients with Minor Injuries

Patients with minor conditions such as sprains and lacerations that require hospital care are triaged to the minor care area. These are patients who will be treated then discharged.

Contaminated Patients

A decontamination area should be set up if the disaster involved a hazardous chemical. Ideally, decontamination is done at the scene by specially trained personnel; however, victims can arrive without benefit of decontamination. These patients pose a risk to personnel caring for them, so preparing the triage team with appropriate clothing and information about the involved material will protect those who come in contact with contaminated patients. Chapter 35: Toxicities provides additional information about toxic exposure.

Table 8-2. Examples of Patient Conditions for Disaster Triage Levels	
Level	**Examples**
Critical	•Airway obstruction, ventilation problems, hemorrhage, comatose patients
Fatal	•Open head injury, crushed skull, crushed chest or torso
Noncritical	•Long-bone fractures, partial or full-thickness burns, major joint dislocation
Minor	•Lacerations, sprains, strains, fractured finger or toe, minor burns

FIELD TRIAGE

Most community disaster plans include use of disaster tags to identify patients at the disaster scene. The tag is torn so the bottom denotes acuity at the scene. Four levels are used. Table 8-3 reviews the specifics of each level. A community may further define each level by the mode of transport. More critical patients may be transported by air or ground ambulance, whereas those with minor injuries may be grouped and transported by bus.

The upper corners of the tag are torn off and left at the scene to indicate where the victim was found. The corner piece may also be placed in locations in crashed planes or buses to tell where the victim was sitting when the crash occurred. Tags have space for noting injuries and other pertinent information. The triage team should read the tag to ascertain this data; however, they must still assess the patient. The field team is working in a hectic, poorly controlled environment and can miss major injuries. The patient's condition can also change between field triage and arrival at the hospital.

Table 3. Field Triage Categories from Disaster Victim Tags		
Color	**Category**	**Description**
Green	Delayed	•Victims with minor wounds who will not suffer complications if left untreated for hours. •Victims who may have mortal wounds in which death appears reasonably certain. •These patients are the last to be transported.
Yellow	Secondary	•Victims who require care but whose conditions are not as life-threatening as first priority victims.
Red	Immediate	•Victims who require immediate attention and transport.
Black	Deceased	•Victims without pulse or respirations who have been in this state for more than 20 minutes or whose injuries make cardiopulmonary resuscitation impossible. •These victims are not transported to the hospital.

SUMMARY

Triage during a disaster is stressful and, exhausting. It requires a level of creativity and flexibility that is rarely necessary in any other situation. Learning the triage role and resource availability before disaster needs arise can minimize anxiety and enhance performance during this unique and, fortunately, rare occurrence.

References

Jordan, K. (Ed.). (2000). <u>Emergency nursing core curriculum</u> (5th ed.). Philadelphia: Saunders.

Kitt, S., Selfridge-Thomas, J., Proehl, J., & Kaiser, K. (1995). <u>Emergency nursing: A physiologic and clinical perspective</u> (2nd ed.). Philadelphia: Saunders.

Joint Commission on Accreditation of Health Care Organizations (JCAHO). (1998). <u>Comprehensive accreditation manual for hospitals: The official handbook</u>. Chicago, IL: Author.

Newberry, L. (Ed.). (1998). <u>Sheehy's emergency nursing: Principles and practice</u> (4th ed.). St. Louis: Mosby.

Learning Assessment Exercises

1. Your facility has initiated the disaster plan in response to a train collision with 200 victims. A set of distressed parents presents to the ED looking for their son who was involved in the train collision. You should:
   a. Have security escort them to their car
   b. Ask them to sit down in the ED waiting area
   c. Ask for their telephone number and then tell them to return home
   d. Ask a volunteer to take them to the hospital lobby

2. Your ED is caring for numerous patients exposed to organophosphate insecticide sprayed from a plane. Members of the news media arrive and begin to take photographs. They also begin to interview you, visitors, and patients. You should:
   a. Answer all of the questions as completely as possible
   b. Ask the ED charge nurse to speak with them immediately
   c. Ignore them and hope they will go away
   d. Contact security or the media relations officer

3. The first patients who arrive from a disaster scene:
   a. Do not require triage unless field triage was not done
   b. Are always the most critically ill or injured patients from the scene
   c. Should be immediately sent to the first available beds in the ED
   d. May require decontamination if a toxic substance is involved in the disaster

4. Which of the following statements is true for triage during a disaster?
   a. Patients with potentially fatal injuries are treated the same during a disaster as during other times.
   b. Triage during a disaster is not performed unless the field team has not completed the triage disaster tag.
   c. All patients are transported to the hospital from the disaster scene.
   d. Disaster management provides care for those with the greatest needs.

1. Review your institution's disaster plan. Identify the role of the ED triage nurse when the plan is activated.

2. Describe management of patients already in the waiting room and triage area when the disaster plan is activated.

3. Review the procedure for patients that come directly to the triage desk during the disaster.

4. Discuss the triage nurse's role in managing patients' family members, visitors, and the media.

5. Review the procedure for patient decontamination.

Clinical Concepts

Clinical Chapters

This section focuses on specific clinical situations that you may encounter as a triage nurse. Completion of these chapters will help you develop skill in triage and assessment of various patient complaints and problems. Chapters are grouped by body area since most subjective complaints lend themselves to this type of categorization. Several complaint categories and specific patient populations are also included. Work with your preceptor to assess patients that fall within each area. With the exception of the chapter on Universal Triage Parameters (Chapter 9) and Advanced Triage Exercises (Chapter 37), chapters are organized alphabetically. Chapters contained in this section are:

- Universal Triage Parameters
- Abdomen/Pelvis
- Abuse and Neglect
- Back
- Bites and Stings
- Burns
- Chest
- Cold-related Conditions
- Confusion
- Ear
- Extremity
- Eye
- Fever
- Head Heat-related Conditions

- Mouth
- Throat
- Neck
- Nose
- Obstetric Complaints
- Psychiatric Complaints
- Respiratory
- Sexual Assault
- Seizure
- Skin Problems
- Surface Wounds
- Toxicities
- Trauma
- Advanced Triage Exercises

The format used for each chapter reflects the triage process—complaint, subjective assessment, objective assessment, diagnostic procedures, interventions, and triage acuity. Information is provided in a bullet format to highlight essential information in the most succinct manner. References are provided for each chapter, but the learner is encouraged to seek other sources to expand their knowledge base.

COMPLAINT - Examples of common complaints for body area or population are provided. These are written as if the patient were voicing the complaint to you. Various levels of patient education and level of understanding were considered when listing complaints. The number of complaints for a each system or category is limitless, but a representative sample of the most common complaints is provided.

SUBJECTIVE ASSESSMENT – Information is listed for the presenting event and the patient history. Historical information includes allergies, medical conditions, prior surgeries, and current medications. The learner is reminded that information may come from the patient, family, caregiver, EMS personnel, police, or various documents.

OBJECTIVE ASSESSMENT – Information obtained during physical assessment is highlighted in this section. Techniques of inspection, auscultation, and palpation are addressed this section.

DIAGNOSTIC PROCEDURES – Ability to order diagnostic tests varies from state to state and facility to facility. Tests listed in this section should serve as a guideline but does not supercede institutional policy and regulatory constraints you may encounter in your specific situation.

INTERVENTIONS – Basic nursing interventions for common patient problems are identified in this section. Your state and/or facility may place limits on specific interventions that can be done by the triage nurse. Follow guidelines established by your facility and state practice act.

TRIAGE ACUITY – Examples of patient complaints or situations that are emergent, urgent, and non-urgent triage acuity are provided. Use these within the context of institutional policy.

Universal Triage Parameters *chapter 9*

OBJECTIVES

After completing this chapter, you will be able to:

1. Identify four parameters assessed for each patient during triage.

2. Describe four interventions that may be routinely implemented in the triage area.

COMPLAINT

- Brief description of what brought the patient to the ED
- Written in the patient's own words when possible

SUBJECTIVE ASSESSMENT

Present Event

- Circumstances surrounding the event
  - What happened
  - Time the event occurred or when symptoms began
  - Treatment prior to arrival and the patient's response to treatment

- Date of last tetanus immunization if there is a wound, burn, abrasion, or foreign body (including in the eye)

- Pain
  - P—What provokes the pain or what palliates (relieves) the pain
  - Q—Quality of the pain (e.g., sharp, burning, pressure, ache)
  - R—Region of pain and radiation of pain
  - S—Severity
  - T—Timing and temporal relation of the pain

History

- All medications routinely taken by the patient
- Any medications taken by the patient in the past 24 hours
- Allergies to medications or latex
- Chronic diseases that may complicate the problem

Trauma

Penetrating Trauma

- Stab wound or impaled object
  - Description of the object
  - Length and width of the object

- Gunshot wound
  - Type of firearm—pellet gun, handgun, rifle, shotgun

-Caliber or mm of the weapon
-Distance between the weapon and the victim

Blunt Trauma
- Motor vehicle crash
  -Type of vehicle—car or truck, small or large
  -Speed of crash and deceleration
  -Patient's location in the vehicle
  -Restraint use—seat belt, air bag, both
  -Point of impact—front, rear, or side
  -Passenger space intrusion
  -Ejection
  -Rollover
  -Ambulatory at scene
  -Outcome of other passengers in vehicle
  -Unusual circumstances (e.g., hit by a train, vehicle fire, found in a river)

- Motorcycle crash
  -Helmet use—full face shield or open face
  -Speed of motorcycle and deceleration
  -Point of impact
  -Distance of ejection
  -Secondary impact
  -Ambulatory at the scene
  -Unusual circumstances

- Accident involving a pedestrian
  -Type of vehicle
  -Speed of vehicle
  -Landing surface
  -Body point of impact
  -Secondary impact
  -Unusual circumstances
  -Thrown into path of second vehicle

- Fall
  -Distance of fall
  -Landing surface
  -Body point of impact
  -Accidental or purposeful
  -Associated problems—alcohol, drugs, gunshot wounds, burns

- Assault or battery
  -Instrument or body part used to inflict injury
  -Areas of body affected

- Boat, jet ski, or snow mobile accident
  -Type of vehicle
  -Circumstances surrounding the crash
  -Point of impact—front, side, rear

-Rollover
-Ejected or run over by the vehicle
-Helmet—full face shield or open face
-Flotation devices
-Other safety equipment
-Associated problems
▪Exposure, delayed rescue from water, others
▪Alcohol or drugs
▪Unusual circumstances—explosion, vehicle sinks, other

OBJECTIVE ASSESSMENT

- Airway, breathing, and circulation (ABCs)

- General skin color, temperature, and moisture

- Level of consciousness

- Vital signs—blood pressure, temperature, pulse, and respirations

- Pulse oximeter if possible respiratory component

DIAGNOSTIC PROCEDURES

- None routinely recommended

INTERVENTIONS

- Provide basic life support for any patient with inadequate ABCs

- Implement cervical immobilization in any patient with blunt trauma if the patient:
-Complains of neck pain
-Has a decreased level of consciousness
-Has been drinking alcohol
-Has sustained a high-impact injury

- Implement appropriate isolation procedures if an infectious disease is suspected

- Administer acetaminophen for fever in infants, children, and adults according to departmental policy

- Provide emotional support to any distressed patient

TRIAGE

Emergent

- Inadequate ABCs

- Unstable vital signs, usually defined in adults as:
-Pulse rate less than 40 or more than 150 beats per minute
-Respiratory rate less than 10 or more than 36 breaths per minute
-Systolic blood pressure less than 80 or more than 200 mm Hg
-Diastolic blood pressure more than 130 mm Hg
-Oxygen saturation less 86%

- Temperature greater than 105 degrees F in an infant or child

- Possible stroke with symptom onset less than 6 hours prior to admission

- Possible myocardial infarction

- Significant mechanism of injury

- Penetrating trauma to the head, neck, chest, abdomen, or groin

- Motor vehicle crash (MVC) with any of the following:
  - High speed—usually greater than 50 mph
  - Change in speed of 20 mph or more
  - Rollover
  - Death in the vehicle
  - Passenger ejected
  - Major vehicle damage

- Two or more proximal long-bone fractures

- Flail chest

- Fall of 20 feet or more

- Pedestrian hit at speed greater than 20 mph

- Burns of the face, airway, or more than 15% body surface area (BSA)

- Severe pain

- Blood and body fluid exposure that is high risk and qualifies for postexposure prophylaxis

Urgent

- Sexual assault with adequate ABCs and no other injuries

- Patient immobilized on a long spine board with no obvious injuries and adequate ABCs

- Reassess every 30 to 60 minutes

Nonurgent

- Adequate ABCs and complaint that does not pose an immediate threat to life, vision or limb (e.g., sore throat, sunburn, constipation)

- Reassess every one to two hours

ESI 5-Level Model

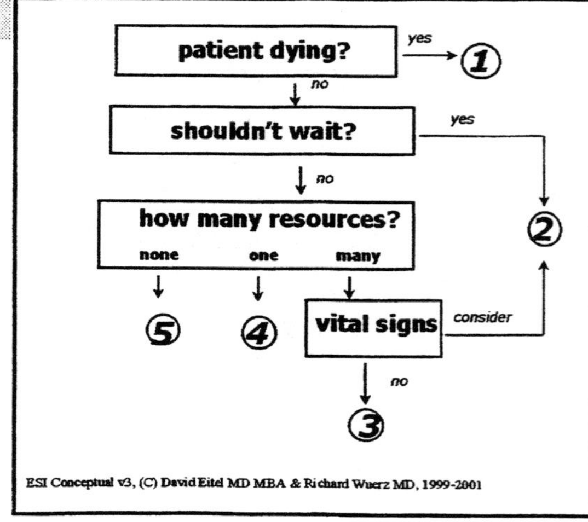

References

Jordan, K. (Ed.). (2000). <u>Emergency nursing core curriculum</u> (5th ed.). Philadelphia: Saunders.

Kidd, P., & Sturt, P. (1996). <u>Mosby's emergency nursing reference</u>. St. Louis: Mosby.

Kitt, S., Selfridge-Thomas, J., Proehl, J., & Kaiser, J. (1995). <u>Emergency nursing: A physiologic and clinical perspective</u> (2nd ed.). Philadelphia: Saunders.

Newberry, L. (Ed.). (1998). <u>Sheehy's emergency nursing: Principles and practice</u> (4th ed.). St. Louis: Mosby.

Rosen, P., & Barkin, R. (1998). <u>Emergency medicine: Concepts and clinical practice</u> (4th ed.). St. Louis: Mosby.

Rosen, P., & Barkin, R., Hayden, S. Shaider, J. & Wolfe, R. (1999). <u>The 5 minute emergency medicine consult</u>. Philadelphia: Lippincott Williams & Wilkins.

1. Cervical spine immobilization should be placed on which of the following patients?
   a. 18 year old male with neck pain for three days unrelated to injury.
   b. 48 year old male who presents to the ED with neck spasms two days after a motor vehicle accident
   c. 35 year old male who fell from the top of a two story building
   d. 51 year old male beaten across the torso with a baseball bat.

2. Immunization history is required on which of the following patients?
   a. Any pediatric patients who do not have a pediatrician
   b. All adult patients
   c. Any patient with break in skin integrity
   d. All patients regardless of complaint

3. The patient is on a long spine board following a minor motor vehicle collision. The patient complains that the board makes his back hurt. He has no obvious injuries and vital signs are within normal limits. What triage acuity should this person receive?
   a. Emergent
   b. Urgent
   c. Non-urgent

4. Date of the patient's last tetanus injection should be determined if the patient has:
   a. Multiple bruises
   b. Corneal abrasion
   c. GI bleeding
   d. Foreign body in the ear

5. Pertinent patient history is related to which of the following:
   a. All medical conditions
   b. Medications taken in the past 24 hours
   c. Any surgical procedures
   d. Any physician caring for the patient in the past month

6. Which of the following patients should receive an emergent acuity rating?
    a. Blood pressure 198/120
    b. Sudden onset left sided weakness
    c. Pulse 116 in a patient with a migraine headache
    d. Red eyes with purulent drainage

7. Which of the following should receive a 5-level rating based on the ESI model?
    a. Active chest pain, shortness of breath
    b. Patient seeking prescription refill
    c. Red eyes with purulent drainage and a temperature of 101 degrees
    d. Blood pressure 198/120

1. Review minimum expectations for triage assessment in your facility.

2. Review triage protocols used in your facility.

3. Identify patient populations not routinely treated in your facility, e.g., pediatrics, obstetrics, trauma. Discuss the procedure should these patients arrive at your door.

Abdomen/Pelvis *chapter 10*

OBJECTIVES

After completing this chapter, you will be able to:

1. Identify four parameters assessed in the patient with a complaint involving the abdomen.

2. Identify three abdominal complaints prioritized as emergent.

COMPLAINT

- Belly hurts
- Stomachache
- Abdominal cramping
- Bloating
- Diarrhea or constipation
- Nausea or vomiting
- Blood in the stool
- Bleeding from the rectum
- Foreign body in the rectum
- Hurts to urinate
- Testicles hurt
- Hurts to have sex
- Bleeding from vagina
- Something stuck in the vagina
- Something stuck in the penis

> **Key Concept**
> Ask the patient to point to where it hurts. The word "stomach" may be used for any part of the abdomen.

SUBJECTIVE ASSESSMENT—ABDOMINAL PAIN
Present Event

- Vomiting
  - Color
  - Frequency
  - Unusual odor

- Location of pain in the abdomen

- Fever

- Upper abdominal or epigastric pain
  - Probable causes include ulcer, liver, and gallbladder problems
  - Does the pain change with eating?
  - How long after eating does pain occur?
  - Do certain foods cause discomfort?
  - Is the patient vomiting?

- Midabdominal pain
  -Probable causes include intestinal problems
  -Vomiting

- Last bowel movement
  -Normal, hard, diarrhea
  -Color
  -Time or date
  -Comparison to normal bowel movements

- Lower abdominal pain
  -Probable causes include reproductive organs and the urinary tract
  -Vaginal discharge or bleeding
    ▪Color
    ▪Amount
    ▪Date of last normal menstrual period
    ▪Odor
    ▪Is the patient sexually active?
    ▪Method of birth control (if any)
    ▪Positive pregnancy test?

- Urinary symptoms
  -Dysuria
  -Frequency
  -Gross hematuria
  -Retention

Key Concept
A patient may menstruate even when pregnant.

History

- Abdominal surgeries

- Clotting disorders

- Aneurysm

- Inflammatory bowel disease

- Pregnancy history
  -Gravida
  -Para
  -Abortions—therapeutic and spontaneous
  -Ectopic pregnancy

- High abdominal, epigastric, or midabdominal pain

- Ulcers, gallbladder or liver disease, pancreatitis

- Alcohol use

- Specific medications (e.g., antibiotics, ulcer medications, aspirin, ibuprofen, steroids, laxatives, anticoagulants)

- Recent abdominal/body piercing

- Lower abdominal pain

- Previous urinary tract infections

- Previous episodes of urinary retention

- Previous pelvic disease

- Exposure to sexually transmitted diseases

- Specific medications (e.g., oral contraceptives, Norplant)

- Other birth control method

SUBJECTIVE ASSESSMENT—DIARRHEA
Present Event
- Frequency

- Stool characteristics
  -Color—bright or dark red
  -Consistency
  -Odor

- Accompanying flatulence

- Is diarrhea explosive?

- Progression of symptoms

- Recent food consumption

- Related abdominal pain

- Recent traveling or camping

- Infants—presence of diaper rash

History
- Usual laxative use (e.g., pills, suppositories)

- Enema use

- Anyone else in household with the same symptoms?

- Significant medications (e.g., laxatives, antidiarrhea medications, anticoagulants, steroids, antibiotics)

SUBJECTIVE ASSESSMENT—VOMITING
Present Event

- Frequency
- Color—red or coffee ground
- Odor—fecal, other
- Time of last meal prior to onset of symptoms
- Fever
- Recent alcohol ingestion
- Last bowel movement
  - Time or date
  - Normal, hard, or diarrhea
- Date of last menstrual period
- Positive pregnancy test

History

- Recent ear infection or dizziness
- Gastrointestinal disorders
- Bowel obstructions
- Recent excessive exercise
- Exposure to extreme heat
- Cancer
- Chemotherapy or radiation therapy
- Recent medications
- Medications that cause nausea (e.g, antibiotics, narcotic analgesics, chemotherapy)
- Irritants (e.g., nonsteroidal anti-inflammatory drugs, digoxin)

SUBJECTIVE ASSESSMENT—RECTAL BLEEDING
Present Event

- Frequency of symptoms
- Color of blood
  - Bright red
  - Dark red
  - Black, tarry stools

> **Key Concept**
> **Bright red blood indicates bleeding in the lower GI tract, whereas tarry stools indicate bleeding from the upper GI tract.**

- Amount

- Recent hard stools

- Recent anal intercourse or penetration with an object

History

- Inflammatory bowel disease

- Ulcers

- Hemorrhoids or fissures

- Routine insertion of objects or anal intercourse

- Weight loss

- Changes in appetite

- Use of alcohol

- Specific medications (e.g., anticoagulants, ulcer medications, aspirin, non-steroidal anti-inflammatory drugs)

SUBJECTIVE ASSESSMENT—DYSURIA OR HEMATURIA
Present Event

- Frequency

- Urgency

- Flank pain

- Back pain

- Radiation of pain

- Fever

- Nocturia or slow, small urination stream

- Progression of symptoms

- Abdominal pain

- Vaginal or penile discharge—color, amount, odor, associated pain

- Males—pain on ejaculation or rectal pain

- Sensation of fullness in lower abdomen

Key Concept
Flank or back pain and fever suggest renal involvement and are more serious than simple urinary tract infections.

History

- Previous urinary tract infections
- Renal calculi
- Enlarged prostate
- Specific medications
- Retention (e.g., anticholinergic medications, antidepressants, antihistamines)
- Dysuria—previous unfinished antibiotic regimen
- Hematuria—beets in diet recently, coumadin

SUBJECTIVE ASSESSMENT—TESTICULAR PAIN
Present Event

- Precipitating event
- Progression of symptoms
- Sudden onset suggests torsion
- Penile discharge
  -Color
  -Amount
  -Dysuria or retention
  -Odor
- Scrotal edema—unilateral or bilateral
- Scrotal redness
  -Lumps or masses in the scrotum
- Fever
- Nausea and vomiting

History

- Inguinal or femoral hernia
- Renal calculi
- Testicular tumor
- Recent infection
- Sexually transmitted disease
- Trauma

SUBJECTIVE ASSESSMENT—VAGINAL BLEEDING/ DISCHARGE AND PENILE DISCHARGE

Present Event

- Abdominal pain

- Fever

- Pain with intercourse

- Bleeding
  -How many pads or tampons used in last hour?
  -Color
  -Clots

- Discharge
  -Color
  -Odor
  -Characteristics—thick, thin, frothy
  -Amount
  -Different from normal discharge

- Dysuria

- Burning or itching

- Sores in perineal area

- Associated itching, bleeding, or discharge from anus

History

- Sexual activity

- Method of birth control (if any)

- Positive pregnancy test

- Pregnancy history
  -Gravida
  -Para
  -Abortions—therapeutic and spontaneous

- Regular or irregular menstrual periods

- Last Pap smear and results

- Specific medications (e.g., anticoagulants, hormones, fertility drugs, antibiotics)

- Discharge

- Known exposure to sexually transmitted disease

- Previous sexually transmitted disease

- Symptoms in partner(s)

- Sexual assault

- Insertion of foreign body into vagina

- Previous infections

- Diabetes

- Cervical cancer

OBJECTIVE ASSESSMENT

- Skin turgor and mucous membranes (dry or moist)

- Color of sclera and skin (if liver or gallbladder disease is suspected)

- Abdominal shape (e.g., concave, flat, distended)

- Areas of tenderness

- Bowel sounds

- Orthostatic vital signs for bleeding, vomiting, or dizziness associated with abdominal symptoms

> **Key Concept**
> **Utilize blood and body fluid precautions for any patient with jaundice.**

DIAGNOSTIC PROCEDURES

- Urinalysis with possible culture and sensitivity

- Blood for complete blood cell count and electrolytes

- Rh and blood type if therapeutic abortion is possible

- Urine or serum pregnancy test

INTERVENTIONS

- None recommended

TRIAGE

Emergent

- Suspected acute abdomen

- Diarrhea with signs of dehydration in a pediatric patient

- Gastrointestinal hemorrhage

- Vaginal hemorrhage

- Urinary retention with painfully full bladder

- Acute onset testicular pain

- Orthostatic hypotension or loss of consciousness when standing

- Significant orthostatic increase in pulse of 40 bpm or more

Urgent

- Moderate abdominal pain

- Diarrhea or vomiting with influenza-like symptoms

- Possible spontaneous abortion with moderate vaginal bleeding and stable vital signs
- Dysuria with fever
- Dark or black rectal bleeding with stable vital signs
- Hematuria in patient taking anticoagulants
- Foreign body in rectum or vagina with related discomfort
- Orthostatic dizziness or pulse increase 20 to 40 bpm

Nonurgent

- Chronic or mild abdominal pain
- Dysuria with no fever
- Vaginal or penile discharge with no abdominal pain
- Chronic diarrhea with no signs of dehydration
- Minimal bright red rectal bleeding
- Recent vomiting or diarrhea without pain or signs of dehydration

ESI 5-Level Model

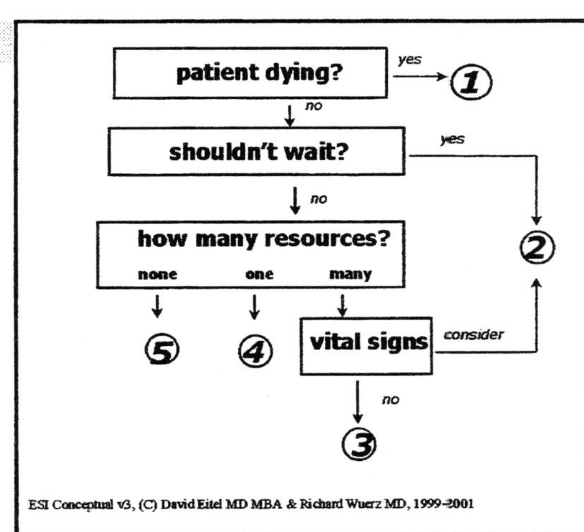

References

Jordan, K. (Ed.). (2000). <u>Emergency nursing core curriculum</u> (5th ed.). Philadelphia: Saunders.

Kidd, P., & Sturt, P. (1996). <u>Mosby's emergency nursing reference</u>. St. Louis: Mosby.

Kitt, S., Selfridge-Thomas, J., Proehl, J., & Kaiser, J. (1995). <u>Emergency nursing: A physiologic and clinical perspective</u> (2nd ed.). Philadelphia: Saunders.

Newberry, L. (Ed.). (1998). <u>Sheehy's emergency nursing: Principles and practice</u> (4th ed.). St. Louis: Mosby.

Proehl, J. (1999). <u>Emergency nursing procedures</u> (2nd ed.). Philadelphia: Saunders.

Rosen, P., & Barkin, R. (1998). <u>Emergency medicine: Concepts and clinical practice</u> (4th ed.). St. Louis: Mosby.

Rosen, P., & Barkin, R., Hayden, S. Shaider, J. & Wolfe, R. (1999). <u>The 5 minute emergency medicine consult</u>. Philadelphia: Lippincott Williams & Wilkins.

1. A clean catch urine specimen should be obtained on which of the following patients:
   a. 35 year old female with vaginal spotting
   b. 30 year old female with burning and frequency
   c. 80 year old male with urinary retention and pain
   d. 47 year old male with severe left flank pain

2. Orthostatic vital signs should be obtained on patients with a complaint (s) of:
   a. High blood pressure – sent from health department
   b. Nausea and vomiting for three days
   c. Intermittent dizziness for 4 months
   d. Sudden onset left flank pain

3. A 65 year old female presents to the ED with severe upper abdominal pain. She is pale, diaphoretic, and has been vomiting dark green emesis. Which of the following objective assessment findings is the most critical to the triage nurse's determination of acuity?
   a. Pale sclera
   b. SBP decreases 40 points with standing
   c. Dry mucous membranes
   d. Hyperactive bowel sounds

4. A 36 year old male complains of sudden onset severe left flank pain. He is diaphoretic and has vomited twice on the way to the hospital. Essential assessment information that should be obtained by the triage nurse includes:
   a. Color of emesis
   b. Color of urine
   c. Level of discomfort
   d. Presence of penile discharge

5. A patient presents with right, lower quadrant abdominal pain, nausea, vomiting, heart rate of 110, and low-grade fever. Based on the ESI 5-Level Model, this patient would be rated at which level?
   a. 1
   b. 2
   c. 3
   d. 4
   e. 5

6. The patient with vaginal bleeding has saturated 10 tampons in the last hour. Which statement applies?
   a. This represents minimal blood loss, so immediate action is not required.
   b. The patient is probably exaggerating the amount of bleeding.
   c. This represents significant bleeding – obtain orthostatic vital signs.
   d. This is not significant information – continue your focused assessment of the complaint.

7. A 12 year old male presents with sudden onset right testicular pain. He walks with his legs bowed and appears to be in severe pain. An emergent triage acuity is given to this patient due to:
   a. Age
   b. Threat to testicular function
   c. Lack of privacy for examination in the triage area.
   d. Psychological Support

8. A 7 year old female is brought to the ED after falling from her bicycle. Which of the following complaints suggests the presence of serious injury?
   a. Abrasions across the knees and elbows
   b. Severe left shoulder pain without obvious sign of injury
   c. Cut on left cheek and laceration of left ear
   d. Fracture left upper arm

1. Review protocols that apply to patients with abdominal pain, urinary complaints, and pain.

2. Discuss placement of patients that require pelvic exams. Identify any specific rooms that are used.

3. Review the most common complaints related to the abdomen which receive care in your facility.

OBJECTIVES

After completing this chapter, you will be able to:

1. Describe three important elements of triage history in the potential abuse victim.

2. Discuss two appropriate interventions the triage nurse can use in caring for potential abuse victims.

3. Describe two elements of triage physical assessment in the potential abuse victim.

RESOURCES

- Policies related to abuse and neglect of children, adults with disabilities, and the elderly; sexual assault; domestic violence; mandatory reporting requirements

INTRODUCTION

Absolute privacy is essential for interviewing and assessing the patient who may have been physically or sexually abused. Triage does not always provide this. If this is the case, obtain chief complaint and perform physical assessment sufficient to determine the patient's condition. Counselors and psychologists trained in interviewing children are best for working with child victims of physical or sexual abuse.

SUBJECTIVE ASSESSMENT—CHILD PHYSICAL ABUSE

Present Event

- Do not make judgments

- Obtain information to direct care and safeguard the patient

- Interview the caretaker separate from a child who is old enough to understand

- Determine the following:
  - When it occurred and what happened
  - Treatment prior to arrival and response to treatment
  - Reasons for any delay seeking health care
  - Recent caretakers of the child other than parents
  - Pre-existing conditions (e.g., blood dyscrasias, bone disorders, hemophilia, disabilities)
  - Other children in the family—location and conditions

Key Concept

Investigate carefully when the history of injury or illness does not match the presenting injuries and symptoms.

OBJECTIVE ASSESSMENT
Bruises, Welts, and Scars

- Buttocks and lower back due to beating
- Genitals, inner thighs, cheeks, and earlobes from slapping or cuffing
- Upper lip and frenulum from forced feedings
- Pressure bruises in the shape of hands or fingertips
- Choke marks
- Bruises in the shape of the instrument used
- Human bite marks anywhere on the body
- Multiple bruises in different stages of healing: Bruises change color as they age
  -Immediate—red marks
  -Zero to 2 days—swollen, tender, red to reddish-purple
  -Two to 5 days—green
  -Five to 7 days—yellow
  -Seven to 10 days—brown
  -Two to 4 weeks—cleared

> **Key Concept**
> **Bruises on soft areas are more suspicious than bruises over bony surfaces.**

Lacerations, Cuts, and Abrasions

- Lips, gums, eyes, and genitals are common sites.
- Human bites may break the skin and can be matched to the perpetrator.

Burns

- Cigarette or match tip burns may be arranged in patterns.
- Contact burns occur from forced contact with heating devices such as an iron or curling iron.
- Forced immersion burns are usually symmetrical with clearly demarcated edges, may be found on limbs or buttocks.

Head Injuries

- Scalp swelling and bruising if child has been struck in the head or thrown against a hard surface.
- Decreased level of consciousness, unilateral motor signs, or pupil changes indicate increased intracranial pressure.
- Unusual injuries to the eyes, ear, nose, and mouth should raise suspicions.
- Hyphemas, corneal abrasions, orbital fractures, and periorbital hematomas are common.

- Shaken baby syndrome usually occurs in infants less than one year old and is associated with altered level of consciousness, seizure, respiratory arrest, and no external signs of trauma.

Abdominal Trauma

- Child exhibits unexplained signs of hypovolemic shock.
- Distended or rigid abdomen with or without bruises may indicate internal bleeding.
- Abdominal pain or persistent vomiting may be present.

Bone and Joint Injuries

- Fresh fractures or multiple fractures in various stages of healing may be present.
- Fractures in an infant less than one year are highly suspicious.

Other Presentations

- Rectal bleeding, hematemesis, seizures, episodes of apnea, diarrhea, vomiting, fever, or rashes that disappear are the most common complaints in Munchausen syndrome by proxy. The child is given large doses of salt, laxatives, emetics, or heavy metals to induce symptoms.

Behavioral Observations

- There may be no behavioral indication of abuse during interactions with the child and caretaker.
- Child may appear withdrawn, have a vacant stare, and make no eye contact.
- Answers in a monotone–flat affect should raise the index of suspicion.
- The child may appear wary of parents and adults, duck at sudden movements, or maintain distance of more than an arm's length.
- The child may stiffen when approached by adults.
- Child may be stoic during painful procedures.
- Regressive behavior (i.e., behaving in a manner too young for age) may be present.

Red Flags for Potential Child Abuse

- Unexplained or unwitnessed injury
- Conflicting story or history inconsistent with injury
- Parent or caretaker hesitates to provide information
- Child is not developmentally capable of causing the described injury
- Inappropriate parental concern—too much or too little
- Delay in seeking health care
- History of repeated suspicious injuries

- Caregiver bypasses hospitals closer to home without reason
- Caregiver seeks care at multiple health care facilities
- Obvious family stressors or social isolation
- Explanation of injury is inconsistent with observed injury
- Parent reluctant to look at or comfort child
- Child is blamed for the injury

INTERVENTIONS

- Determine interventions for the presenting complaint and initial treatment indicated by the assessment.
- Ensure the ABCs and initiate other interventions as appropriate.
- Remember that the abuser may not be the parent or caregiver. It may be a baby-sitter, relative, or other caretaker. When this occurs, the parent or caregiver may arrive in a highly emotional state. Provide privacy and offer support.
- Document subjective and objective assessment, including verbatim parent or caregiver comments.
- Routinely take photos of any injuries. Refer to your specific departmental policy.
- Report suspicions to the appropriate investigative agency. Refer to your department policy for further assistance.

SUBJECTIVE ASSESSMENT—CHILD SEXUAL ABUSE

Presenting Event

- Acute or chronic sexual abuse
- Description of sexual acts that occurred
- Location of the incident(s)
- Date(s) and time(s) of incident(s)
- Name of perpetrator if known, relation to child, and current location
- Threats, bribes, intimidation, physical force, or other violent activity
- Involvement of other adults and children
- Sexual acting out with siblings, peers, or adults
- Preoccupation with sexual matters
- Excessive masturbation
- Regressive behavior
- Enuresis and/or encopresis
- Sleep disorders or nightmares
- Excessive fears

- Suicidal behavior or signs of depression
- Alcohol or other drug abuse
- Change in school performance
- Promiscuity, prostitution, and running away
- History of physical or sexual abuse

OBJECTIVE ASSESSMENT

- Trauma of genitals or rectum
- Vaginal, penile, or rectal lacerations
- Presence of foreign secretions
- Vaginal bleeding or discharge
- Penile bleeding or discharge
- Foreign bodies in the vagina, rectum, or urethra
- Vaginal pain or itching
- Rectal pain or itching
- Urinary tract infection—dysuria
- Sexually transmitted diseases
- Pregnancy

> **Key Concept**
> **There may be no physical signs of sexual abuse.**

INTERVENTIONS

- Similar to those for physical abuse

SUBJECTIVE ASSESSMENT—BATTERED ADULT PRESENTING EVENT

- Nature of the injury
- Circumstances surrounding the event
- When and where it occurred
- What happened
- Treatment prior to arrival
- Previous episodes of domestic violence or abuse
- Crying about minimal injuries
- Unreasonable defensiveness or anger
- Minimizing the seriousness of injuries

- Overly attentive, controlling, or defensive partner, spouse, or caregiver
- Lack of eye contact or fearful eye contact
- Nervous or inappropriate laughter

OBJECTIVE ASSESSMENT

Physical Abuse

- Bruises, welts, scars
- Strangulation marks
- Lacerations, cuts, puncture wounds, abrasions to face, chest, or abdomen—especially if patient is pregnant
- Eye and ear injuries
- Fractured nose
- Head injuries from direct blow or from head being driven into a solid object
- Bilateral injuries sustained when facing attacker head on
- Bruising or fractures of ulnar surfaces when arms were held up to defend head
- Multiple injuries in various stages of healing
- Human bites
- Injuries of breast, abdomen, and genitals in pregnant patient
- Miscarriage due to injury

Psychological Trauma

- Hyperventilation
- Heart palpitations
- Headache
- Choking sensations
- Chest pain
- Hypertension
- Gastrointestinal disturbances
- Suicidal attempts
- Sleep disorders
- Eating disorders
- Self-mutilation
- Self-induced abortions

Other Forms of Abuse

- Forced sexual intercourse or other forced sexual acts
- Pregnancy in a comatose individual or an adult who is severely disabled
- Social isolation

- Home imprisonment
- Economic deprivation
- Verbal harassment

SUBJECTIVE ASSESSMENT—ELDER ABUSE
Presenting Event

- Nature of the injury
- Circumstances surrounding the event
- When and where it occurred
- What happened
- Treatment prior to arrival
- Previous episodes of abuse
- Minimizing the seriousness of injuries
- Overly attentive or controlling caregiver
- Lack of eye contact or fearful eye contact
- Delayed treatment
- Exaggerated defensiveness from caretaker
- Hostility toward patient by caretaker
- Vague explanation or denial in face of injury
- Refusal to discuss problems or injuries with caretaker or in caretaker's presence
- Afraid of caretaker
- Signing legal documents when the patient is not capable of understanding the documents
- Failure to meet basic needs despite adequate resources
- Misappropriation of funds, stolen money, or valuables
- Inadequate heating or cooling

OBJECTIVE ASSESSMENT

- Multiple injuries, burns, or bruises
- Dehydration
- Malnutrition, persistent hunger
- Over- or undermedicated
- Poor hygiene
- Lack of essential medical attention
- Hip and proximal femur fractures
- Multiple untreated or poorly treated decubitus ulcers
- Untreated physical or mental health problems
- Genital bruising or lacerations

Red Flags of Adult Abuse

- Vague history that does not match injuries
- Delay between time of injury and seeking treatment
- Overprotective family members who do not allow the suspected victim alone with the triage nurse
- Repeated ED visits with injuries becoming more severe as frequency increases
- Minimizing the injuries by the suspected victim
- Repeated chronic injuries
- Belittling patient by partner or family or stating the patient is clumsy or stupid

INTERVENTIONS

- Determine interventions depending on presenting complaint and patient acuity
- Consider separating the caregiver and patient if you suspect abuse
- Document injuries with photographs as directed by your facility
- Report the incident to legal authorities as required in your state

TRIAGE

Emergent

- Unstable vital signs
- Hemorrhage or other life-threatening injuries
- Severe emotional distress

Urgent

- Sexual assault with adequate ABCs and no other injuries

Nonurgent

- Minor bruises and lacerations

References

Jordan, K. (Ed.). (2000). <u>Emergency nursing core curriculum</u> (5th ed.). Philadelphia: Saunders.

Kidd, P., & Sturt, P. (1996). <u>Mosby's emergency nursing reference</u>. St. Louis: Mosby.

Kitt, S., Selfridge-Thomas, J, Proehl, J. & Kaiser, J. (1995). <u>Emergency nursing: A physiologic and clinical perspective</u> (2nd ed.). Philadelphia: Saunders.

Newberry, L. (Ed.). (1998). <u>Sheehy's emergency nursing: Principles and practice</u> (4th ed.). St. Louis: Mosby.

Rosen, P., & Barkin, R. (1998). <u>Emergency medicine: Concepts and clinical practice</u> (4th ed.). St. Louis: Mosby.

Strange, G., Ahrens, W., Schafermeyer, R., & Toepper, W. (1999). <u>Pediatric emergency medicine: A comprehensive study guide</u>. New York: McGraw-Hill.

Rosen, P., & Barkin, R., Hayden, S. Shaider, J. & Wolfe, R. (1999). <u>The 5 minute emergency medicine consult</u>. Philadelphia: Lippincott Williams & Wilkins.

1. Determine which of the following statements is true or false about abuse and neglect.

   There are physical and behavioral indications of abuse.

   Nurses are not responsible for identifying possible abuse.

   One hallmark of abuse is incompatibility between history given and the injury observed.

   Remove the parent immediately from the child's room if you suspect abuse or neglect.

2. List five red flags for potential child abuse.
   -
   -
   -
   -
   -

3. Name five common injuries that may be associated with child abuse.
   -
   -
   -
   -
   -

4. Identify five behaviors that may be observed in the abused child.
   -
   -
   -
   -
   -

5. Elder abuse is suspected in an 80 year old male brought to the ED. The most likely perpetrator of this abuse is:
    a. A stranger
    b. Neighbor
    c. Occasional visitor
    d. Caretaker

6. Elder abuse is characterized by:
    a. Financial abuse
    b. Psychological abuse
    c. Physical abuse
    d. All the above

1. What aspects of the patient interview should be completed by the triage nurse when abuse or neglect is suspected?

2. Describe strategies that can be used to maintain a therapeutic environment for the child and the caregiver in situations of suspected child abuse.

3. Discuss abuse and neglect in the following patient populations.

   a. Elderly patients

   b. Infants and children

   c. Disabled adults

   d. Spouses/Domestic partners

OBJECTIVES

After completing this chapter, you will be able to:

1. Describe two parameters assessed for the patient with complaints of back pain.

2. Identify two back conditions that are prioritized as emergent.

COMPLAINT

- Back pain
- Back hurts
- Back spasms
- Hurt back when lifting
- Can't move back
- Back has gone out
- Knot on back
- Swelling on the back

SUBJECTIVE ASSESSMENT

Present Event

- Events surrounding onset of pain
- Known trauma
- Mechanical reason for fall or injury
- Presence of foreign body or wounds in the back
- Medical reason such as syncope, cardiac, or neurologic symptoms
  -Chapter 36: Trauma discusses trauma of the back and spine.
  -Refer to other appropriate chapters for discussion of medical reasons.
- No known trauma
- Abdominal pain
- Fever or chills
- Dysuria or urinary retention
- Groin pain
- Motor or sensory changes
- Syncope or dizziness
- Bladder function
- Bowel function

History

- Previous back injury or surgery

- Degenerative disk disease

- Tumor of spine or metastatic disease

- Cardiovascular disease or hypertension

- Thoracic or abdominal aneurysm

Key Concept
Abdominal or thoracic aneurysm can present as back pain. Assess cardiovascular status carefully if pain radiates from back to front or front to back.

- Last normal menstrual period

- Previous pulmonary embolus

- Previous pulmonary problems—pleuritis or pneumonia

- Specific medications (e.g., analgesics, muscle relaxers, birth control pills, cardiovascular medications, steroids)

- Previous treatment (e.g., hot, cold, exercises, massage, acupuncture, acupressure, chiropractic, other)

OBJECTIVE ASSESSMENT

- Posture and ability to sit and stand

- Gait

- Grip strength or lower extremity strength

- Sensory function of lower extremities

- Point tenderness over vertebrae

- Tenderness over costovertebral angles

- Redness or swelling of painful area

- Pulses in upper and lower extremities if aneurysm known or suspected

Key Concept
Place the patient in spinal immobilization if there is any concern based on mechanism of injury.

DIAGNOSTIC PROCEDURES

- Urinalysis if dysuria or related symptoms

INTERVENTIONS

- Provide mobility assistance—wheelchair or stretcher as appropriate
- Provide ice pack for blunt trauma—rotate on and off every 20 minutes

TRIAGE

Emergent

- Mid to high back pain associated with abdominal pain and hypotension or other signs of cardiovascular compromise
- Low back pain with unilateral or bilateral radiation, perineal anesthesia, motor weakness of the lower extremities, and bowel or bladder dysfunction
- Acute motor or sensory deficits
- Low back pain in patient with lower extremity deficits, bowel or bladder deficits, and history of tumor, vertebral fracture, disk herniation, abscess, or hematoma

Urgent

- Low back pain with vaginal bleeding and possible pregnancy
- Back or flank pain with fever or chills

Nonurgent

- Minor back pain that is localized
- Chronic back pain with or without minor exacerbation and no neurovascular deficits
- Back pain associated with flu symptoms, fever, and myalgia

References

Jordan, K. (Ed.). (2000). <u>Emergency nursing core curriculum</u> (5th ed.). Philadelphia: Saunders.

Kidd, P., & Sturt, P. (1996). <u>Mosby's emergency nursing reference</u>. St. Louis: Mosby.

Kitt, S., Selfridge-Thomas, J., Proehl, J., & Kaiser, J. (1995). <u>Emergency nursing: A physiologic and clinical perspective</u> (2nd ed.). Philadelphia: Saunders.

Newberry, L. (Ed.). (1998). <u>Sheehy's emergency nursing: Principles and practice</u> (4th ed.). St. Louis: Mosby.

Rosen, P., & Barkin, R. (1998). <u>Emergency medicine: Concepts and clinical practice</u> (4th ed.). St. Louis: Mosby.

Rosen, P., & Barkin, R., Hayden, S. Shaider, J. & Wolfe, R. (1999). <u>The 5 minute emergency medicine consult</u>. Philadelphia: Lippincott Williams & Wilkins.

1. Select the most appropriate statement for use of ice for a back injury.
    a. Use the ice pack continuously for the first four hours after injury.
    b. Use ice continuously beginning 24 hours after the injury.
    c. Use the ice pack over the injured area for 24 hours after injury with 20 minutes of ice followed by 20 minutes without ice.
    d. Alternate ice pack application with heat application for the first 24 hours after the injury.

2. Surgical intervention is required within six hours to prevent permanent paralysis and bladder dysfunction in which of the following conditions:
    a. Rheumatoid arthritis
    b. Spinal cord compression
    c. Sciatica
    d. Acute disc rupture

3. Severe back pain frequently occurs in all the following situations except:
    a. Aortic dissection
    b. Menstrual pain
    c. Labor
    d. Appendicitis

4. Point tenderness over the costovertebral angle suggests a problem with the:
    a. Aorta
    b. Pancreas
    c. Kidneys
    d. Spine

5. Which of the following statements about spinal immobilization applied by the triage nurse is true?
    a. A soft cervical collar is used.
    b. Apply spinal immobilization if the patient has an injury and complains of neck pain.
    c. Immobilization can be applied after the patient is taken by wheelchair to the treatment area.
    d. The patient may walk to the treatment area with the collar in place.

6. Determine the most appropriate priority for the following patients.

   a. A 69 year old male presents to the ED with moderate to severe back pain on the left side. He describes a burning sensation that started with a rash. He has been unable to sleep for several days.

   b. A 42 year old female presents with left flank pain and dysuria for four days. She is pale and has an oral temperature of 103 F. She has had nausea and vomiting for two days.

   c. A 12 year old male comes to the ED after falling from the roof of his house and landing on his feet. He complains of severe ankle pain and mid back pain. He is unable to ambulate due to ankle pain and says his legs are tingling. He denies neck pain or loss of consciousness.

   d. A 62 year old female presents with a history of breast cancer and spinal metastases. She complains of back pain and weakness in the lower extremities. She is unable to walk and has not voided in 12 hours. She increased her dose of long acting opioid four hours before arrival, but the pain has only worsened.

   e. A 48 year old male complains of moderate to severe lower back pain. He rates the pain as 6 on the pain scale of 0–10. Pain apparently started after he lifted a microwave oven. He walks slowly with slightly flexed knees.

   f. A 15 year old adolescent presents with left posterior rib pain after his younger sister jumped from the sofa onto his back. He has guarded respirations with increasing dyspnea. His color is pale and his respiratory rate is 34 per minute.

   g. A 56 year old female requests a muscle relaxant for neck and shoulder spasms related to arthritis. She is visiting for the holidays and forgot her medications at home.

   h. A 24 year old female was kicked by a horse in the right posterior ribs while falling off the animal. She is dyspneic and extremely pale. Her pulse is 140 bpm. She denies loss of consciousness.

1. Review the procedure for getting patients with back pain out of the car if this is required in your facility.

2. Review the policy for application of spinal immobilization in patients injured hours or days before arrival.

3. Identify location of equipment for spinal immobilization in your facility. Describe appropriate technique for application of the cervical collar, head-blocks/neck rolls, long spine board, and tape.

Bites and Stings *chapter 13*

OBJECTIVES

After completing this chapter, you will be able to:

1. Identify three potentially lethal bite injuries.

2. Discuss two interventions for bite and sting injuries.

COMPLAINTS

- Stung by a wasp
- Stung by a bee
- Bit by a dog
- Bit by a cat
- Bit by a person
- Bit by a bat
- Bit by an animal—not sure what kind
- Stung by a jellyfish

- Snake bite
- Bit by a rattlesnake
- Bit by a copperhead
- Bit by a coral snake
- Spider bite
- Stung by a scorpion
- Bit by a Gila monster
- Bit by a fire ant

SUBJECTIVE ASSESSMENT
Presenting Event

- Circumstances surrounding the bite or sting
- Mechanism of injury—identity of creature causing the injury
- Animal bite
- Insect bite or sting
- Spider bite—black widow and brown recluse spiders are the most toxic
- Human bite
- Snake bite

> **Key Concept**
> **Human bites are more prone to infection because of oral contaminants.**

- Location on body
- Contamination of wound
- Estimated blood loss
- Change in sensation or motor ability
  -Chapter 19: Extremity describes assessment of extremity problems

- Color, temperature, and moisture of affected area
- Itching, pain, or numbness of the site and surrounding tissue
- Systemic symptoms
- Difficulty breathing
- Weakness, dizziness, or headache
- Nausea and vomiting
- Sensory or motor changes
- Muscle spasms
- Animal bite
- Domestic or wild animal
- Behavior of animal
- Provocation of bite
- Current location of animal
- Animal's immunization status if known

Key Concept
The honeybee stings only once, whereas yellow jackets, wasps, and other hymenoptera sting repeatedly. Stings are cumulative—the greater the number of stings, the greater the reaction.

History
- Known allergy to the sting
- Family history of allergic reactions to stings
- Previous treatment with antivenin
- Previous treatment with rabies prophylaxis
- Hemophilia or other disorders that are associated with bleeding
- Immune disorders such as diabetes that are associated with delayed healing
- Specific medications (e.g., anticoagulants, steroids)

Key Concept
Pit viper venom (from rattlesnakes, copperheads, and water moccasins) is primarily hemotoxic, whereas coral snake venom is primarily neurotoxic.

OBJECTIVE ASSESSMENT
- Type of wound—laceration, abrasion, avulsion, or crush
- Description of the wound—length, depth, shape, and location

- Location of the wound
- Characteristics—irregular, complex, tissue appearance, gaping
- Contamination and presence of foreign bodies
- Discoloration—red, ecchymotic, black center
- Fang, bite, or puncture marks
    - Signs of envenomation (see Table 13-1)
- Edema of surrounding tissue
- Associated hives, rash, or swelling
- Petechiae
- Work of breathing
- Dyspnea
- Decreased oxygen saturation
- Abnormal breath sounds (e.g., wheezing, stridor)

Table 13-1. Signs of Envenomation

None	Fang marks only. No local or systemic reactions noted.
Minimal	Fang marks present. No systemic reaction noted, but local swelling and pain are present.
Moderate	Fang marks are present. Swelling is progressing beyond the area of the bite. Systemic reactions such as nausea, vomiting, and hypotension are present.
Severe	Fang marks are present. There is marked swelling and subcutaneous ecchymosis of the extremity. Severe systemic symptoms such as coagulopathy are present.

Laskowski-Jones, L. (2000). Responding to summer emergencies. *Dimensions of Critical Care Nursing, 19*(4), 2-12.

> **Key Concept**
> **Children are more likely to sustain severe facial bites from dogs and other large animals because of their size in relation to the animal's mouth.**

DIAGNOSTIC PROCEDURES

- None recommended

INTERVENTIONS

- Place insect or snake in a fang-proof container and do not open the container.
- Remove rings or constricting items from the involved extremity.

For insect bites with no systemic reaction

- Apply an ice pack to the area, rotate on and off every 20 minutes
- Remove stingers by scraping

For snake bites

- Draw an indelible line along edge of redness and swelling
- Measure circumference of the affected limb
- Support limb at or below the level of the heart
- Remove any ice packs
- Do not apply tourniquets
- Remove any tourniquets applied by the patient if vascular compromise is present
- Notify animal control according to local guidelines
- Do not dispose of a reptile in the plumbing or trash

**Key Concept
Use caution even if the snake is dead.
Movement can occur up to 24 hours.**

TRIAGE

Emergent

- Signs of anaphylaxis
- Sting or venomous bite with systemic reactions
- Snake bite with rapid swelling
- Seizures

Urgent

- Tissue necrosis, depending on location
- Infected wound
- Local reaction with history of systemic reactions
- Multiple stings

Nonurgent

- Punctures, abrasions, and mild or no cellulitis
- Local reaction with no previous history of systemic reactions
- Known nonvenomous snake bite with local reaction

References

Jordan, K. (Ed.). (2000). <u>Emergency nursing core curriculum</u> (5th ed.). Philadelphia: Saunders.

Kidd, P., & Sturt, P. (1996). <u>Mosby's emergency nursing reference</u>. St. Louis: Mosby.

Kitt, S., Selfridge-Thomas, J., Proehl, J., & Kaiser, J. (1995). <u>Emergency nursing: A physiologic and clinical perspective</u> (2nd ed.). Philadelphia: Saunders.

Laskowski-Jones, L. (2000). Responding to summer emergencies. <u>Dimensions of Critical Care Nursing, 19</u>(4), 2-12.

Newberry, L. (Ed.). (1998). <u>Sheehy's emergency nursing: Principles and practice</u> (4th ed.). St. Louis: Mosby.

Rosen, P., & Barkin, R. (1998). <u>Emergency medicine: Concepts and clinical practice</u> (4th ed.). St. Louis: Mosby.

Rosen, P., & Barkin, R., Hayden, S. Shaider, J. & Wolfe, R. (1999). <u>The 5 minute emergency medicine consult</u>. Philadelphia: Lippincott Williams & Wilkins.

1. Children have a greater risk for reaction to bites and stings because:
   a. They are outside more than adults are so they are more likely to be stung.
   b. There is a smaller volume in which venom is distributed so concentration is stronger.
   c. The child's immune system has not fully developed.
   d. Children wear bright colors so they are more likely to attract more than one insect.

2. Human bites are more likely to become infected because:
   a. Skin reacts quickly to contaminants in the mouth.
   b. There are a large number of contaminants in the mouth.
   c. Teeth drive saliva deep into tissues with human bites.
   d. There is a strong antigen-antibody reaction between humans.

3. A patient presents with multiple stings from a honeybee. Which of the following statements applies?
   a. The stings are from one or two honey bees.
   b. The stings are from many bees.
   c. The reaction does not increase with the number of stings.
   d. Multiple stings can cause anaphylaxis with the first exposure to the venom.

4. Children are more likely to sustain facial bites from dogs and other large animals because:
   a. Children are more likely than adults to hug these animals.
   b. The child's size places the face closer to the animal's mouth.
   c. Clothing protects the child from other injuries.
   d. Lack of subcutaneous fat in the child's face.

5. A patient presents with severe swelling after a bite from an unknown snake. This swelling suggests the bite was due to:
   a. Allergic reaction to the snake venom
   b. Venom was from a coral snake
   c. Venom was from a pit viper
   d. Crush injury from the snake bite.

6. A patient comes to the ED with the snake that bit him. The triage nurse should:
   a Open the container to identify the snake.
   b. Make sure the container is fang-proof.
   c. Place the snake on ice to minimize risk of movement after death.
   d. Ask the patient to take the snake to the car then return for treatment.

1. Identify poisonous snakes and spiders indigenous to your practice area.

2. Discuss resources available to you for identification of poisonous snakes.

3. Review the procedure for management of anaphylaxis in the triage area.

4. Discuss protocols that apply to anaphylaxis, management of bites and stings, or reporting specific injuries.

5. Review local guidelines for rabies prophylaxis and reporting animal bites.

Burns *chapter 14*

OBJECTIVES
After completing this chapter, you will be able to:

1. Identify three types of burns.

2. Describe three signs of airway involvement in the burned patient.

COMPLAINT
- Burns from flame, steam, hot liquid, or hot object

- Sunburn

- Electrical burn

- Cough or trouble breathing after exposure to smoke or toxic fumes

- Burns or skin irritation from a chemical

- Chemical contamination or possible exposure

SUBJECTIVE ASSESSMENT
Present Event
- Type of burn
  -Thermal
  -Chemical
  - Form—liquid, powder, or gas
  - Identity, if known
  -Electrical
  -Radiant

- Circumstances surrounding the burn

- Enclosed space

- Explosion

- Duration of exposure

- Body area affected
  -Chapter 20: Eye discusses thermal and chemical eye injuries.

- Inhalation

- Heated air or steam

- Smoke

- Toxic fumes

History

- Asthma or other respiratory problems
- Conditions that impair healing—diabetes, immune disorders
- Tetanus immunization status
- Specific medications (e.g., steroids, bronchodilators if inhalation injury)

OBJECTIVE ASSESSMENT

- Signs of airway involvement
- Facial burns or swelling
- Singed facial or nasal hair
- Carbon, soot, chemical in mouth, nose, or sputum
- Decreased ability to swallow or handle secretions
- Dyspnea
- Hoarseness or vocal changes
- Critical location—face, hands, feet, perineum, or overlying major joints
- Circumferential burns of the digits, extremities, neck, or chest
- Extent of burn in percentage of body surface area (BSA)
- Depth of burn—superficial partial thickness, deep partial thickness, or full thickness
- Evidence of chemical on skin or clothes
- Circulation, motor function, and sensation distal to burned extremity

DIAGNOSTIC PROCEDURES

- None recommended

INTERVENTIONS

- Remove jewelry and constrictive clothing
- Apply cool, moist sterile compresses to small burns for comfort; avoid ice
- Moderate elevation of extremities
- Decontaminate according to department protocol
- Prevent spread of chemical contamination
- Administer tetanus prophylaxis per department protocol
- Offer emotional support

TRIAGE

Emergent

- Respiratory or airway involvement

- Significant electrical burns

- Chemical burns or contamination

- Partial-thickness burns greater than 20% BSA

- Full-thickness burns greater than 10% BSA

- Deep partial- or full-thickness burns of face, hands, feet, perineum, or overlying major joints

- Burns with concomitant injury

Urgent

- Partial-thickness burns 10 to 20% BSA

- Full-thickness burns 2 to 10% BSA

Nonurgent

- Partial-thickness burns less than 10% BSA

- Full-thickness burns less than 2% BSA

- Minor skin irritation after chemical exposure and decontamination

- Superficial sunburn

References

Jordan, K. (Ed.). (2000). <u>Emergency nursing core curriculum</u> (5th ed.). Philadelphia: Saunders.

Kidd, P., & Sturt, P. (1996). <u>Mosby's emergency nursing reference</u>. St. Louis: Mosby.

Kitt, S., Selfridge-Thomas, J., Proehl, J., & Kaiser, J. (1995). <u>Emergency nursing: A physiologic and clinical perspective</u> (2nd ed.). Philadelphia: Saunders.

Newberry, L. (Ed.). (1998). <u>Sheehy's emergency nursing: Principles and practice</u> (4th ed.). St. Louis: Mosby.

Rosen, P., & Barkin, R. (1998). <u>Emergency medicine: Concepts and clinical practice</u> (4th ed.). St. Louis: Mosby.

Rosen, P., & Barkin, R., Hayden, S. Shaider, J. & Wolfe, R. (1999). <u>The 5 minute emergency medicine consult</u>. Philadelphia: Lippincott Williams & Wilkins.

1. An acuity rating of non-urgent should be given to which of the following patients?
   a. 17 year old who splashed grease on the left arm and hand.
   b. 30 year old female with burn to anterior thigh from spilled soup.
   c. 2 year old who is hoarse after drinking hot coffee
   d. Adult male who says he was knocked to the ground by lightning.

2. Which of the following assessment findings suggests airway involvement in the patient burned in a house fire?
   a. Deep circumferential burns of the chest and abdomen
   b. Concurrent electrical injury
   c. Cyanotic nail beds
   d. Singed nasal hairs.

3. Pertinent historical data for the patient with a thermal burn includes:
   a. Stopped smoking 12 months ago
   b. History of diabetes
   c. Occasional alcohol use
   d. History of hypertension

4. A patient presents with severe blistering of the hand following exposure to a hot liquid. The most appropriate action for the triage nurse is:
   a. Determine name of primary care physician.
   b. Wrap hand in ice pack.
   c. Place hand below level of the heart.
   d. Remove jewelry immediately.

5. Pertinent medical history for the patient with severe burns of the torso and lower extremities secondary to a brush fire includes:
   a. Takes vitamins every day
   b. Fracture left femur 2 years ago
   c. Insulin dependent diabetic
   d. Last meal 16 hours ago

Clinical Application

1. Discuss management of burn patients in your facility. Identify resources for burn care in the community.

2. Identify applicable protocols for the burn patient, e.g. tetanus prophylaxis, wound care, pain management.

Chest *chapter 15*

OBJECTIVES

After completing this chapter, you will be able to:

1. Discuss four parameters assessed on patients who complain of chest pain.

2. Identify a patient with chest pain who should receive an emergent priority rating.

COMPLAINT

- Chest pain
- Chest feels funny
- Left arm pain
- Heart beating too fast
- Heart beating funny
- Palpitations
- Pacemaker not working
- AICD is firing
- Chest is jumping

SUBJECTIVE ASSESSMENT—CHEST PAIN

Present Event

- Pain
  - -Worse on inspiration or movement
  - -Point tenderness that can be reproduced with palpation

- Pain quality
  - -Crushing
  - -Sharp
  - -Dull
  - -Constant
  - -Comes and goes

- Pain characteristics
  - -Radiates to arm, shoulders, neck, jaw, or back
  - -Alleviating factors
    - ▪Rest
    - ▪Position
    - ▪Eating or not eating
    - ▪Medications such as nitroglycerine, analgesics, and antacids
    - ▪Cough
    - ▪Painful
    - ▪Productive or dry

- Hemoptysis

- Shortness of breath, dyspnea on exertion, or orthopnea

- Nausea and vomiting

- Diaphoresis

- Dizziness or syncope

- Anxiety or feeling of doom

- Pallor

- Palpitations

Key Concept
Patients with diabetes and other neuropathies may not present with classic chest pain symptoms.

History

- Cardiac history

- Myocardial infarction(s) (MI)

- Angina

- Dysrhythmia

- Implanted pacemaker

- Implanted cardiac defibrillator

- Cardiac surgery

- Congestive heart failure

- Aneurysm

- Congenital defects

- Atherosclerotic heart disease

- Cardiac risk factors

- Family history

- Smoking

- Hypertension

- Diabetes

- Hypercholesterolemia

- Usual exercise habits

- Recent stress, illness, or exertional activity

- Recent trauma

- Recent respiratory infection

- Recent intravenous drug use

- Ulcer disease or hiatal hernia

- Specific medications (e.g., anticoagulants, cardiac medications, antihypertensives, hypoglycemics, insulin, cocaine, amphetamines)

SUBJECTIVE ASSESSMENT—HEART BEATING FAST/SLOW/IRREGULAR OR PALPITATIONS

Present Event

- Pain (as above)

- Dyspnea

- Weakness, dizziness, syncope

- Precipitating event

- New medicines

- Ingestion of substances (e.g., cocaine, amphetamines, caffeine)

- Exposure to carbon monoxide

History

- Heart disease, angina, previous MI, or rhythm disturbances

- Heart valve disorder—mitral valve prolapse

- Hypertension

- Cardiac medications with any recent change in dosage or medication

- Decongestants, antihistamines, or other stimulants

OBJECTIVE ASSESSMENT

- Airway patency

- Stridor

- Ability to speak

- Muffled voice or grunting

- Respirations

- Work of breathing

- Ability to speak full sentences

- Splinting or guarding

- Bilateral chest wall movement

- Chest deformity

- Favored position

- Retractions

- Respiratory pattern

- Capillary refill time

- Jugular vein distension

- Pedal edema

- Oxygen saturation decreased

- Pallor or cyanosis

- Diaphoresis

DIAGNOSTIC PROCEDURES

- Electrocardiogram

- Pulse oximetry if respiratory component

INTERVENTIONS

- Administer oxygen

- Transport by wheelchair to decrease oxygen demand

> **Key Concept**
> **Cardiac-related chest pain is not age-specific. Increasing levels of stress, recreational drug use, diet medications, and other causative factors have widened the age span for those who may experience an MI.**

TRIAGE

Emergent

- Respiratory distress

- Chest pain with ischemic cardiac characteristics

Urgent

- Point tenderness with normal vital signs, oxygen saturation, and no associated symptoms

ESI 5-Level Model

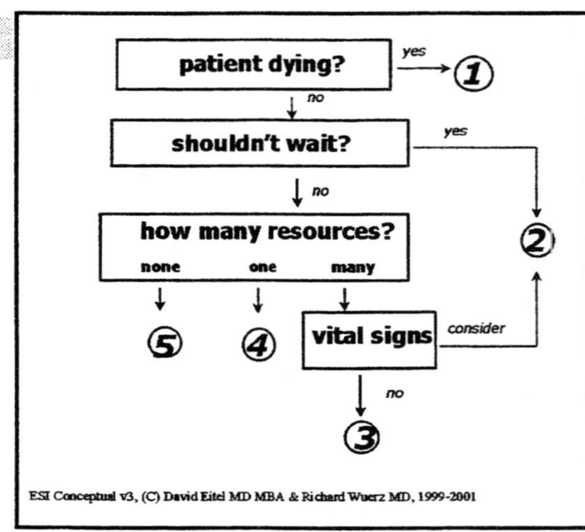

References

Jordan, K. (Ed.). (2000). <u>Emergency nursing core curriculum</u> (5th ed.). Philadelphia: Saunders.

Kidd, P., & Sturt, P. (1996). <u>Mosby's emergency nursing reference</u>. St. Louis: Mosby.

Kitt, S., Selfridge-Thomas, J., Proehl, J., & Kaiser, J. (1995). <u>Emergency nursing: A physiologic and clinical perspective</u> (2nd ed.). Philadelphia: Saunders.

Newberry, L. (Ed.). (1998). <u>Sheehy's emergency nursing: Principles and practice</u> (4th ed.). St. Louis: Mosby.

Rosen, P., & Barkin, R. (1998). <u>Emergency medicine: Concepts and clinical practice</u> (4th ed.). St. Louis: Mosby.

Rosen, P., & Barkin, R., Hayden, S. Shaider, J. & Wolfe, R. (1999). <u>The 5 minute emergency medicine consult</u>. Philadelphia: Lippincott Williams & Wilkins.

1. A complaint of indigestion that may be related to a cardiac problem is suggested by pain that:
   a. Is positional
   b. Is relieved by antacids
   c. Radiates to the left shoulder
   d. Always happens after eating fast food.

2. A 45 year old male presents to the ED with substernal chest pain, diaphoresis, and shortness of breath. The most appropriate triage acuity for this patient is:
   a. Emergent
   b. Urgent
   c. Nonurgent

3. Which of the following statements is considered true for the classic picture of pain associated with myocardial infarction?
   a. Pain radiates to the neck, jaw, arm, or back.
   b. Medical problems such as diabetes do not affect presentation of pain.
   c. The younger the patient, the less likely they are to have a classic picture of pain.
   d. Females always present with the classic picture of pain related to an MI.

4. A patient presents to the ED with severe chest pain. Which assessment finding represents critical information?
   a. Skin is damp but warm
   b. History of cocaine abuse
   c. Pain is constant and goes straight through to the back.
   d. Had a normal EKG two weeks prior to arrival.

5. A 48 year old patient presents to the ED with weakness. What is your most appropriate course of action?
   a. Determine the patient's surgical history
   b. Identify the patient's private physician.
   c. Take the patient's pulse
   d. Obtain the patient's temperature.

6. A patient enters with shortness of breath, mild to moderate respiratory distress, and oxygen saturation of 91%. Based on the ESI 5-Level Model, this patient would be at which level?
   a. 1
   b. 2
   c. 3
   d. 4
   e. 5

1. Review applicable chest pain protocol for your facility.

2. Identify the location of the nearest crash cart.

3. Discuss management of a cardiac arrest in triage.

4. Review management of cardiac arrest on the ambulance ramp and in adjacent parking lots if appropriate.

5. Determine the shortest route from triage to the treatment area for patients with chest pain.

OBJECTIVES

After completing this chapter, you will be able to:

1. Identify two cold-related emergencies that should be prioritized as emergent.

2. Describe two interventions for the patient with a cold-related emergency.

COMPLAINT

- Frostbite
- Frozen fingers or toes
- Patient found outside in cool or cold environment
- Elderly patient with altered level of consciousness in a cool or cold environment

- Exposure
- Frozen
- Found in water

> **Key Concept**
> Hypothermia is not limited to cold northern climates. Submersion in water can also lead to hypothermia. Heat loss is 25 to 32 times greater in water than in air.

SUBJECTIVE ASSESSMENT

Present Event

- Possible hypothermia
- Conditions present when patient was found (e.g. location-inside, outside, in water)
- Estimated temperature of the environment
- Clothing or covering—wet or dry
- Estimated length of exposure
- Evidence of alcohol or drug ingestion
- Injuries
- Possible frostbite
- Area of involvement
- Duration of exposure
- Protective clothing
- Digits thawed, then frozen again
- Pain or sensation

History

- Medical conditions
- Adrenal failure or sepsis
- Hypopituitary disease
- Hypothyroidism
- Hypoglycemia
- Alterations in mental status
- Specific medications (e.g., alcohol, barbiturates, phenothiazines, narcotics, stimulants, heroin)

OBJECTIVE ASSESSMENT

- Level of orientation
- Confused, flat affect, poor judgment
- Affected tissue
  -Hard, malleable, or soft
  -Color
- Capillary refill
- Wounds
- Pain

> **Key Concept**
> **Loss of the ability to shiver is a indication of significant hypothermia.**

- Core temperature of 90 to 95 degrees F
  -Shivering, lethargy, and/or confusion
  -Bradycardia or tachycardia with occasional atrial fibrillation
- Core temperature of 87 to 90 degrees F
  -Generalized rigidity and/or coma
  -Hypoventilation
  -Bradycardia and/or increased myocardial irritability
  -Hypovolemia and blood sludging
  -Shivering impaired
- Core temperature of less than 87 degrees F
  -Shivering absent
  -Coma, areflexia, and/or fixed and dilated pupils
  -Apnea and/or cyanosis
  -Bradycardia, ventricular fibrillation, and asystole

DIAGNOSTIC PROCEDURES

- None recommended

INTERVENTIONS

- Remove wet clothing and cover with a dry, light blanket

- Gently wrap frozen digits in dry sterile gauze

TRIAGE

Emergent

- Core temperature of less than 92 degrees F

- Frozen digits

Urgent

- Core temperature of 92 to 95 degrees F with normal mental status

Nonurgent

- Core temperature above 95 degrees F and normal mental status

ESI 5-Level Model

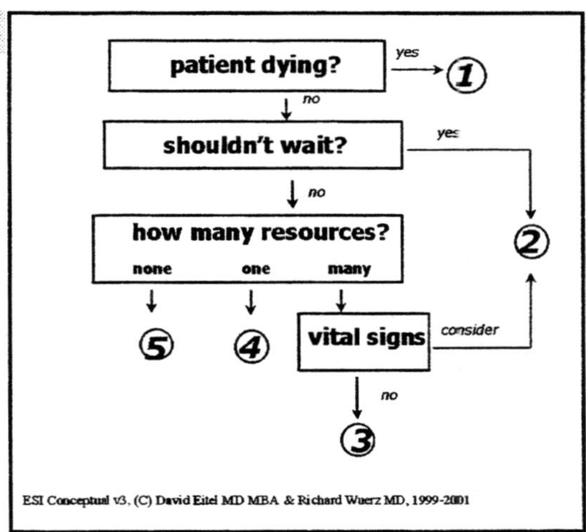

References

Jordan, K. (Ed.). (2000). <u>Emergency nursing core curriculum</u> (5th ed.). Philadelphia: Saunders.

Kidd, P., & Sturt, P. (1996). <u>Mosby's emergency nursing reference</u>. St. Louis: Mosby.

Kitt, S., Selfridge-Thomas, J., Proehl, J., & Kaiser, J. (1995). <u>Emergency nursing: A physiologic and clinical perspective</u> (2nd ed.). Philadelphia: Saunders.

Newberry, L. (Ed.). (1998). <u>Sheehy's emergency nursing: Principles and practice</u> (4th ed.). St. Louis: Mosby.

Rosen, P., & Barkin, R. (1998). <u>Emergency medicine: Concepts and clinical practice</u> (4th ed.). St. Louis: Mosby.

Rosen, P., & Barkin, R., Hayden, S. Shaider, J. & Wolfe, R. (1999). <u>The 5 minute emergency medicine consult</u>. Philadelphia: Lippincott Williams & Wilkins.

1. A patient is found unconscious on the ground. The patient skin is cold. Which of the following items listed on a medical alert bracelet should increase your index of suspicion for hypothermia?
   a. Blood thinners
   b. Diabetes
   c. Hypertension
   d. Pacemaker

2. Which of the following patients is at greater risk for hypothermia?
   a. 16 year old with temperature 91 degrees Fahrenheit
   b. 10 month old carried into the ED without a blanket
   c. 44 year old unconscious with cold skin who does not shiver
   d. 69 year old without heat for six hours

3. Loss of body heat increases significantly with:
   a. Advanced age
   b. Thin clothing
   c. Pre-existing heart disease
   d. Immersion in water

4. The most significant indicator for hypothermia is:
   a. Loss of ability to shiver
   b. Cold extremities
   c. Bradycardia
   d. Hypotension

5. Medical conditions that place the patient at risk for hypothermia include:
   a. Hyperthyroidism
   b. Diabetic ketoacidosis
   c. Salicylate toxicity
   d. Sepsis

6. Medications that place the patient at risk for hypothermia **do not** include:
   a. Amphetamines
   b. Ethanol
   c. Heroin
   d. Phenothiazines

1. Review protocols for management of hypothermia in your facility.

2. Identify warming appliances and/or procedures available to you in the triage area.

3. Identify the lowest reading for the thermometer in the triage area.

4. Review the previous patient descriptors and categorize each based on the 5-level triage system.

CONFUSION *chapter 17*

OBJECTIVES

After completing this chapter, you will be able to:

1. Identify two diagnostic tests indicated for the confused patient.

2. Identify three patients who should be prioritized as emergent.

COMPLAINT

- Forgets things
- Loss of inhibitions
- Not acting "right"
- Memory loss
- Unable to perform activities of daily living
- Going "downhill"
- Incontinent of stool or urine
- Keeps getting lost
- Confused
- Agitated

SUBJECTIVE ASSESSMENT
Present Event

- Progression of symptoms—acute or chronic
- Circumstances surrounding onset of symptoms
- Loss of consciousness
- Memory loss
- Sudden or gradual onset
- Changes in elimination habits
- Nausea, vomiting, or diarrhea
- Other fluid losses
- Headache—location, severity, and radiation
- Preceding events
- Recent trauma
- Recent illness
- Fever
- Associated muscle weakness
- Changes in gait
- Changes in speech

History

- Significant medical conditions
- Stroke or transient ischemic attacks
- Diabetes
- Seizures
- Renal failure, dialysis
- Liver disease
- Head injury, tumors, or surgeries
- Hypertension
- Alcoholism or other drug addiction
- HIV status
- Recent change in medications or dosages
- Recent discharge from the hospital or nursing home
- Similar symptoms in the past
- Workup for dementia or Alzheimer's disease
- Home situation
- Lives alone or with family
- Community resources

OBJECTIVE ASSESSMENT

- Oxygen saturation
- Grip strength
- Facial asymmetry
- Potential for violence
- Level of orientation
- General appearance
- Skin turgor
- Poor personal hygiene
- Bizarre attire
- Clothing inappropriate for weather
- Picking at hair or clothes
- Associated injuries

Key Concept
Ischemic stroke management with intravenous thrombolytic agents must be done within three hours of onset of symptoms. Assume that there is a medical cause for confusion until probable causes have been ruled out.

DIAGNOSTIC PROCEDURES

- Finger stick glucose (serum glucose)
- Serum and urine for drug tests
- Breath alcohol test if available
- Serum electrolytes

INTERVENTIONS

- Defuse potential violence
- Control violent behavior
- Monitor whereabouts if confused

TRIAGE

Emergent

- Confusion with new onset changes in speech or gait
- Confusion with fever
- Confusion with seizures
- Confusion with history of brain surgery, head injury, or tumor
- Harmful to self or others

Urgent

- Chronic confusion with acute changes

Nonurgent

- Chronic confusion with no acute changes

References

Jordan, K. (Ed.). (2000). <u>Emergency nursing core curriculum</u> (5th ed.). Philadelphia: Saunders.

Kidd, P., & Sturt, P. (1996). <u>Mosby's emergency nursing reference</u>. St. Louis: Mosby.

Kitt, S., Selfridge-Thomas, J., Proehl, J., & Kaiser, J. (1995). <u>Emergency nursing: A physiologic and clinical perspective</u> (2nd ed.). Philadelphia: Saunders.

Newberry, L. (Ed.). (1998). <u>Sheehy's emergency nursing: Principles and practice</u> (4th ed.). St. Louis: Mosby.

Rosen, P., & Barkin, R. (1998). <u>Emergency medicine: Concepts and clinical practice</u> (4th ed.). St. Louis: Mosby.

Rosen, P., & Barkin, R., Hayden, S. Shaider, J. & Wolfe, R. (1999). <u>The 5 minute emergency medicine consult</u>. Philadelphia: Lippincott Williams & Wilkins.

1. Critical historical information for an 80 year old patient with new onset confusion includes:
   a. Jaundice for two days
   b. Urinary retention for 12 hours
   c. Atrial fibrillation treated with coumadin
   d. Hyperthyroidism

2. New onset confusion in an 86 year old patient with bipolar disorder may be the result of:
   a. Normal manifestation of bipolar changes
   b. Expected presentation of bipolar disorder in the elderly
   c. Physiologic changes of aging
   d. An unidentified medical condition

3. A 42 year old female who is 18 weeks pregnant with her first child is brought to the ED with severe loss of memory. The most appropriate diagnostic test in triage is:
   a Fetal heart tones
   b. Urinalysis
   c. Orthostatic vital signs
   d. Finger stick glucose

1. Review indications for fingerstick glucose test in triage.

2. Discuss management of suspected stroke patients in your facility.

OBJECTIVES

After completing this chapter, you will be able to:

1. Describe three parameters assessed on the patient with an ear problem.

2. Discuss two interventions for the patient with ear pain.

COMPLAINT

- Earache
- Bleeding or drainage
- Can't hear
- Ears stopped up
- Decreased hearing
- Ringing in ears
- Dizziness or room spinning
- Pulling at ears
- Blow to ear
- Ears plugged
- Put something in his or her ear
- Bug in the ear
- Paper in the ear
- Foreign body in the ear
- Buzzing in ears
- Chemical in ear

SUBJECTIVE ASSESSMENT
Present Event

- Fever
- Drainage—color and amount
- Pain
  -Onset and character
  -Ear pain and/or headache
  -Worse with chewing or movement of tragus or pinna
- Upper respiratory infection
- Dizziness—onset and character
- Nausea and/or vomiting
- Crying or fussy infant
- Tinnitus or hearing changes
- Facial swelling and/or redness

Key Concept
Severe pain just before ear drainage begins is associated with a ruptured tympanic membrane.

History

- Previous ear infections
- Presence of polyethylene tubes and age when inserted
- Other ear surgeries
- Prior need for ear irrigation
- Frequent swimming or diving
- Menière's disease
- Labyrinthitis
- Motion sickness
- Regular use of earphones, earplugs, or earmuffs
- Stuck something in the ear
- Salicylate overdose

OBJECTIVE ASSESSMENT

- Visible foreign body
- Red and/or swollen external ear
- Redness and/or swelling of ear canal
- Visible cerumen impaction
- Wounds or sores of external ear or ear canal
- Drainage
  -Unilateral or bilateral
  -Color and amount
- Pain—duration and severity
- Crying, restless, or fussy infant
- Bulging tympanic membrane

DIAGNOSTIC PROCEDURES

- Test fluid for glucose when drainage is associated with head trauma.

Key Concept
Clear ear drainage that is positive for glucose contains cerebrospinal fluid and is associated with a basilar skull fracture.

INTERVENTIONS

- Use an ice pack if external trauma
- Provide warm, moist compresses if no history of injury
- Provide acetaminophen for fever or pain
- Provide tetanus prophylaxis if wound present

TRIAGE

Emergent

- Tinnitus associated with salicylate overdose
- Severe pain

Urgent

- Live insect or foreign body that is likely to swell in the ear
- Drainage from ear with related head injury
- Ringing in ears with dizziness
- Hearing changes with dizziness
- Severe nausea and vomiting associated with vertigo

Nonurgent

- Uncomplicated mild earache
- Inanimate foreign body that is not likely to swell
- Drainage with minimal associated complaints
- Tinnitus with minimal associated complaints

References

Jordan, K. (Ed.). (2000). <u>Emergency nursing core curriculum</u> (5th ed.). Philadelphia: Saunders.

Kidd, P., & Sturt, P. (1996). <u>Mosby's emergency nursing reference</u>. St. Louis: Mosby.

Kitt, S., Selfridge-Thomas, J., Proehl, J., & Kaiser, J. (1995). <u>Emergency nursing: A physiologic and clinical perspective</u> (2nd ed.). Philadelphia: Saunders.

Newberry, L. (Ed.). (1998). <u>Sheehy's emergency nursing: Principles and practice</u> (4th ed.). St. Louis: Mosby.

Proehl, J. (1999). <u>Emergency nursing procedures</u> (2nd ed.). Philadelphia: Saunders.

Rosen, P., & Barkin, R. (1998). <u>Emergency medicine: Concepts and clinical practice</u> (4th ed.). St. Louis: Mosby.

Rosen, P., & Barkin, R., Hayden, S. Shaider, J. & Wolfe, R. (1999). <u>The 5 minute emergency medicine consult</u>. Philadelphia: Lippincott Williams & Wilkins.

1. A patient presents to the ED with a chief complaint of ringing in the ears. Which of the following statements warrants giving this patient an emergent priority?
   a. Hit in the ear with an open hand
   b. Severe sinus headache
   c. Tubes inserted in ear two weeks prior to arrival
   d. Child ate a jar of Ben-Gay ointment

2. The most appropriate priority for a patient who has a bug in the left ear is:
   a. Emergent
   b. Urgent
   c. Non-urgent

3. Risk for ear infections increases with:
   a. Tubes inserted before the age of 12 months
   b. Use of cotton swabs
   c. Previous episode of otitis media
   d. Frequent swimming

4. A 5-month-old is brought to the ED crying loudly. There is no drainage but the child is pulling at both ears. Which of the following statements contributes to the triage nurse's determination of acuity?
   a. Infants less than 6 months of age do not develop severe ear infections
   b. Lack of drainage rules out the possibility of a severe ear infection
   c. Temperature should be ascertained before priority is assigned.
   d. Pediatric patients experience significant pain with an ear infection

5. A 27 year old female presents to the ED complaining of a mild earache. Pain started 24 hours ago. Pertinent historical information includes swimming daily in a nearby lake. What is the most appropriate triage acuity for this patient?
   a. Emergent
   b. Urgent
   c. Non-urgent

6. Serous drainage with mild to severe ear pain suggests which of the following problems?
   a. Bulging tympanic membrane
   b. Foreign body in the ear
   c. Infection
   d. Drug toxicity

1. Discuss comfort measures for ear pain that can be applied in the triage area.

2. Discuss ear irrigation as a triage intervention if appropriate for your facility.

3. Discuss insect extraction as a triage intervention if appropriate.

Extremity *chapter 19*

OBJECTIVES

After completing this chapter, you will be able to:

1. Identify three assessment parameters for patients with swollen joints.

2. Describe three complaints that should receive an emergent priority.

COMPLAINT

- Leg or arm hurts
- Leg or arm swollen
- Pain in joints
- Hurts to move arm or leg
- Arthritis
- Gout
- Rubbing sound when wrist moves
- Foreign object in joint (e.g., nail, stick, wire, other)

- Cut off finger(s) or toe(s)
- Puncture wound
- Shoulder out of joint
- Dislocated finger, shoulder, knee
- Broken finger, hand, wrist, arm
- Broken toe, foot, ankle, leg
- Injured arm or leg

> **Key Concept**
> Life-threatening musculoskeletal problems are the result of hemorrhage, multisystem injury, and/or fat embolism.

> **Key Concept**
> Musculoskeletal injuries may be associated with any life-threatening injuries. Treat threats to life before treating an extremity problem.

SUBJECTIVE ASSESSMENT

Present Event

- Known trauma
- Position of extremity at time of injury—inversion, eversion, extension, flexion, rotation
- Mechanical reason for fall or injury (e.g., tripped, stepped in hole, hit by a car)
- Medical reason—syncope, cardiac, or neurologic symptoms
- Associated sounds—popping, cracking
- Ability to move, use, or bear weight since injury
- No known trauma

- Progression of symptoms

- Repetitive movement of area

- Systemic problems

- Fever or chills

- Shortness of breath or dyspnea on exertion

- Refer to Chapter 32: Skin Problems for discussion of skin and soft tissue complaints.

- Refer to Chapter 13: Bites and Stings for discussion of bite injuries.

- Refer to Chapter 36: Trauma for discussion of severe extremity trauma.

> **Key Concept**
> **Limb-threatening musculoskeletal problems are caused by disruption of vascular supply and/or neurologic innervation.**

History

- Previous injury or surgery in area of complaint

- Occupational or recreational factors—computer use, sports, others

- Pregnancy

- Unrelated illness or injury during past several weeks (e.g., strep throat, rheumatic fever)

- Chronic conditions

- Hemophilia

- Sickle cell disease

- Arthritis

- Cardiac disease

- Stroke

- Seizure

- Peripheral neuropathy

- Motor or sensory deficits

- Diabetes

- Cancer

- Paget's disease

- Renal disease

- Osteoporosis

- Gout

- Joint pain

- Intravenous drug use

- Gonococcal infection

- Previous treatment—splints, bandages, heat, cold, massage, chiropractic, acupressure, acupuncture

- Tetanus immunization status

- Specific medications (e.g., anticoagulants, steroids, cardiac medications, oral contraceptives)

OBJECTIVE ASSESSMENT

- Presence and degree of deformity

- Abnormal positioning

- Guarding injured area

- Swelling or tenseness of skin over muscle compartments

- Discoloration—erythema, pallor, ecchymosis

- Surface trauma—open wound in area of deformity, bone protrusion, abrasions

- Pedal edema—amount and presence of pitting

- Breath sounds and pulse oximetry if dyspnea is present

- Crepitus or hematoma in area of injury

- Gentle range of motion

- Palpate and evaluate the five Ps (see Table 19-1)

- Foreign object—type and location
    - Bleeding or pulsation associated with object
    - Entrance and exit wounds

> **Key Concept**
> Neurologic assessment may be unreliable in the patient with pre-existing paralysis, neuropathy, cold exposure, or prior consumption of analgesics.

Table 19-1. Five Ps of Extremity Assessment

Parameter	Description
Pain	•Note point of maximal tenderness. Palpate distal to this area and move proximally. Include joint above and below the painful area. •Palpate for point tenderness. •Palpate the "anatomical snuffbox" for navicular pain in wrist injuries.
Pulses	•Note pulse presence and strength distal to the injury. •Assess capillary refill distal to the injury. •Compare capillary refill and pulses bilaterally.
Pallor	•Observe color distal to injury. Compare bilaterally. •Compare color and temperature bilaterally, proximally, and distally.
Paralysis	•Assess motor function of the affected limb.
Paresthesia	•Determine whether sensation is normal, decreased, or absent distal to injury.

DIAGNOSTIC PROCEDURES

- X-ray to rule out fracture, dislocation, subluxation, or foreign body

INTERVENTIONS

- Splint painful area or place in position of comfort
- Remove potentially constrictive clothing and jewelry
- Elevate injured extremity when possible
- Apply ice pack for 20 minutes followed by 20 minutes without the ice pack
- Stabilize foreign object
- Provide tetanus prophylaxis if wound is present

TRIAGE

Emergent

- Impaired neurovascular function
- Uncontrolled bleeding
- Increased pain with passive range of motion
- Significant increase in pain since crush injury, surgery, or cast application
- Traumatic limb amputation
- Pedal edema with respiratory distress
- Significant crush injury

Urgent

- Patient with medical reason for fall or injury
- Dislocation without neurovascular compromise
- Joint injury in patient with hemophilia
- Bone deformity without neurovascular compromise
- Joint pain with fever
- Patient appears ill or toxic
- Possible fracture with bleeding disorder or anticoagulant therapy
- Calf or leg pain with dyspnea and/or cough
- Extensive or grossly contaminated wound

Nonurgent

- Minor extremity injury without deformity or swelling
- Ongoing joint pain with history of repetitive stress or forceful motion of part
- Localized joint pain or swelling without fever

References

Jordan, K. (Ed.). (2000). <u>Emergency nursing core curriculum</u> (5th ed.). Philadelphia: Saunders.

Kidd, P., & Sturt, P. (1996). <u>Mosby's emergency nursing reference</u>. St. Louis: Mosby.

Kitt, S., Selfridge-Thomas, J., Proehl, J., & Kaiser, J. (1995). <u>Emergency nursing: A physiologic and clinical perspective</u> (2nd ed.). Philadelphia: Saunders.

Newberry, L. (Ed.). (1998). <u>Sheehy's emergency nursing: Principles and practice</u> (4th ed.). St. Louis: Mosby.

Rosen, P., & Barkin, R. (1998). <u>Emergency medicine: Concepts and clinical practice</u> (4th ed.). St. Louis: Mosby.

Rosen, P., & Barkin, R., Hayden, S. Shaider, J. & Wolfe, R. (1999). <u>The 5 minute emergency medicine consult</u>. Philadelphia: Lippincott Williams & Wilkins.

1. A patient presents to the ED with severe left calf pain. The patient denies pre-existing medical problems but states the pain started yesterday after his leg was caught between two cars. The most appropriate triage action is:
   a. Apply ice
   b. Elevate the leg
   c. Assess pulses
   d. Place in position of comfort

2. A patient arrives in the ED with deformity of the left forearm. The patient states the injury occurred during a fall off the roof. Priority action for the triage nurse is:
   a. Splint the arm and apply an ice pack
   b. Immobilize the person's cervical spine
   c. Determine allergies and medical history
   d. Obtain vital signs

3. Which of the following statements about temporary splints is NOT true?
   a. The splint should extend one joint above and one joint below the injury.
   b. The splint can be made of anything rigid enough to support the extremity.
   c. The splint should be removed as soon as the patient arrives at the ED.
   d. The splint is applied by one person while the injured part is supported by another.

4. A 16 year old male presents to the ED 24 hours after application of a fiberglass cast to his right arm from the hand to above the elbow. The patient complains of numbness and tingling in his hand and fingers. The most likely cause of this problem is:
   a. The patient's age.
   b. Short time since cast application.
   c. Use of fiberglass casting material.
   d. Circulatory compromise from the cast.

5. A 17 year old female presents to the ED with severe swelling and pain of the right wrist. What historical information is NOT pertinent to assessment of the complaint?
   a. The patient had a fracture of left wrist at the age of ten.
   b. The patient injects recreational intravenous drugs.
   c. The patient has sickle cell disease.
   d. The patient is pregnant.

6. A 55 year old male presents to the ED with an 18 inch metal spike through his left foot. The most appropriate first action for the triage nurse is:
   a. Transport the patient immediately to the treatment area.
   b. Stabilize the metal spike.
   c. Remove the patient's shoe and sock.
   d. Place betadine soaked gauze on the skin at the point of entry.

7. A 78 year old patient presents with severe pedal edema. What assessment is critical for the triage nurse to determine patient acuity?
   a. Temperature
   b. Weight
   c. Pulse oximetry
   d. Circumference of both calves

8. All the following patient situations should receive a triage acuity of emergent except:
   a. Joint pain with fever 100.4 °F.
   b. Amputation left hand
   c. Crush injury right calf
   d. Pulse is diminished below obvious fracture.

1. Review the splinting options used in the triage area for upper and lower extremities.

2. Determine the most appropriate mode of transportation from the triage area to the treatment area for patients with severe extremity injuries.

3. Discuss the procedure for getting patients with lower extremity injuries out of cars.

4. Identify the location for ice or ice packs in the triage area.

EYE *chapter 20*

OBJECTIVES

After completing this chapter, you will be able to:

1. Test visual fields.

2. Test visual acuity.

3. Identify two eye complaints that require an emergent priority.

COMPLAINT

- Pink eye
- Red eye
- Swollen
- Painful
- Draining
- Itching
- Tearing
- Sensitive to light
- Change in vision
- Double vision
- Curtain vision
- Red vision
- Flashing lights
- Foreign body in eye
- Stye or boil on eyelid
- Pupils not equal
- Unable to remove or locate contact lens
- Cut
- Burn
- Welding burns
- Blood in eye
- Scratched eye
- Hit in eye
- Punctured eye
- Poked in eye
- Something in eye
- Chemical splashed in eye

SUBJECTIVE ASSESSMENT
Present Event

- Eye affected—left, right, or both
- Vision changes
- Blurring
- Diplopia
- Loss of vision—gradual or sudden
- Flashing lights, floaters, or curtain over eyes
- Red or brown vision
- Yellow vision—usually associated with digoxin toxicity
- Pain—sudden and severe or gradual and moderate

- Vision correction
  - Contact lens
    - Hard or soft lenses
    - Are lenses in place now?
  - Glasses

- Trauma

- What part of eye was injured?

- Protective eyewear used
  - Wearing glasses or contact lenses when incident happened?

- Motor vehicle collision
  - Did air bag deploy or explode?

- Chemical exposure
  - Name of chemical if available (do not waste time trying to identify the chemical)
  - Irrigation prior to arrival
  - Chemical spilled on other body areas or clothing

- Medical conditions
- Progression of symptoms
- Recent sinus infection or upper respiratory infection

History

- Previous eye problems
- Previous rough visual acuity
- Glaucoma
- Eye surgeries
- Lens implant
- Diabetes or hypertension
- Tetanus immunization status
- Specific medications (e.g., anticoagulants, topical ophthalmic medications, digoxin)
- Occupation (e.g., welder, works with lasers)
- Others in household or people who have contact with patient have the same complaint

Key Concept
Conjunctivitis is contagious.

OBJECTIVE ASSESSMENT

- Test visual acuity

- Use the Snellen chart

- Check each eye then both eyes simultaneously

- Check if the patient is or is not wearing glasses or contact lens

- Have the patient count the number of fingers

Key Concept
Use a visual acuity chart appropriate for age and reading ability. Charts are available with multiple letters, the letter "E", or easily recognized shapes.

- Do not forcefully open the eye

- Palpate orbit and surrounding bony structures if there has been blunt trauma to orbit

- Test visual fields

- Inspect for tissue integrity

- Inspect cornea for clarity, disruption, visible foreign body, redness, or layer of blood

- Check pupil shape, size, and reactivity

- Assess color of sclera and conjunctiva

- Look for edema or redness of lids or periorbital area

- Check discharge color and consistency

- Determine tenderness, crepitus, or anesthesia

DIAGNOSTIC PROCEDURES

- None recommended

INTERVENTIONS

- Immobilize visible penetrating foreign body immediately to prevent further injury.

- Apply cool packs for swelling or comfort unless the globe is perforated or there is evidence of other penetrating injury.

- Elevate the head 45 to 90 degrees F if there is leakage of aqueous humor, the cornea is red, or there is blood in the anterior chamber.

- Instill ophthalmic anesthetic if a foreign body is not associated with signs of infection or globe penetration.

- Begin irrigation immediately for chemical injury to the eye.

- Administer tetanus prophylaxis per facility protocol.

> **Key Concept**
> Emergent eye problems are the second greatest threat recognized by the triage nurse—after threats to life and before threats to limb.

TRIAGE

Emergent

- Sudden loss of vision
- Diminished loss of vision with pain
- Sudden severe eye pain
- Alkaline or acid chemical exposure
- Impaled or penetrating foreign body
- Suspected globe laceration or rupture
- Suspected hyphema
- Tears of the iris

Urgent

- Periorbital swelling with fever
- Visual change in patient with history of glaucoma
- Blurred or double vision after trauma
- Severe lid wounds

- Subconjunctival hemorrhage without pain or vision loss

- Vague, minor, or chronic eye pain

- Clear or crusty drainage from eyes

- Gradual change in vision

- Soft tissue swelling or ecchymosis without vision changes

- Nonpenetrating foreign body

- Ptosis without trauma

References

Jordan, K. (Ed.). (2000). <u>Emergency nursing core curriculum</u> (5th ed.). Philadelphia: Saunders.

Kidd, P., & Sturt, P. (1996). <u>Mosby's emergency nursing reference</u>. St. Louis: Mosby.

Kitt, S., Selfridge-Thomas, J., Proehl, J., & Kaiser, J. (1995). <u>Emergency nursing: A physiologic and clinical perspective</u> (2nd ed.). Philadelphia: Saunders.

Newberry, L. (Ed.). (1998). <u>Sheehy's emergency nursing: Principles and practice</u> (4th ed.). St. Louis: Mosby.

Proehl, J. (1999). <u>Emergency nursing procedures</u> (2nd ed.). Philadelphia: Saunders.

Rosen, P., & Barkin, R. (1998). <u>Emergency medicine: Concepts and clinical practice</u> (4th ed.). St. Louis: Mosby.

Rosen, P., & Barkin, R., Hayden, S. Shaider, J. & Wolfe, R. (1999). <u>The 5 minute emergency medicine consult</u>. Philadelphia: Lippincott Williams & Wilkins.

1. Visual acuity should NOT be done before treatment for which of the following patients:
   a. Sudden loss of vision in left eye
   b. Eye pain after poked in eye
   c. Drain cleaner splashed in eyes
   d. Red eyes with drainage

2. You suspect globe rupture in a patient with trauma to left eye. What is your next action?
   a. Apply cool packs for comfort, to control bleeding, and decrease orbital edema.
   b. Order x-rays of the affected orbit to rule out foreign body or orbit fracture
   c. Gently lift orbit to evaluate pupil reaction to light.
   d. Transport immediately to the treatment area.

3. A non-urgent priority should be given to which of the following patients?
   a. Adult male with swelling around the left eye – possibly caused by an insect bite a day or so ago. Oral temperature is 101.2 F
   b. Eight month old infant with recent upper respiratory infection. Presents with low grade fever and purulent drainage from both eyes.
   c. Adult female who suddenly noted blood in the lower lateral aspect of the right eye. The patient has no history of trauma, previous eye problems, or chronic health problems. The patient denies pain.
   d. Adult male with a sensation of something in his eye since cleaning a brush pile earlier in the day. His eye is red and tearing.

4. Determine triage acuity for the following patients.

Triage Acuity	Patient Information
___________	54 year old female complains of new onset headache which is severe and crushing. Her speech is slurred and she has an unsteady gait.
___________	34 year old male arrives with a laceration of the left upper eyelid that extends beyond the eyebrow. There is no bleeding or apparent involvement of the globe. Visual acuity is normal.
___________	19 year old female presents with watery, itching eyes off and on for two weeks. Temperature is 98.4 F. The patient is eating a sandwich and states she must be back at work in 5 minutes.
___________	10 month old male with a two-day history of upper respiratory infection and bilateral purulent eye drainage. The infant is playing quietly in his mother's lap. Temperature is normal.

20 year old male struck on the right side of the face with a base ball. He complains of blurred vision and tenderness over the lower orbit. No hyphema is noted.

____

4 year old male is brought to the ED crying and rubbing his eyes. Thirty minutes prior to arrival, someone sprayed an unknown household cleaner in the child's face. Conjunctiva and surrounding skin are red. Child does not cooperate with gross visual acuity.

____

1. Locate Snellen charts for the triage area. Confirm the 20 foot mark where the patient will stand.

2. Review guidelines for eye irrigation in the triage area.

3. Determine location of supplies for eye irrigation in the triage area.

4. Discuss protocols for management of eye problems including triage instillation of topical anesthetics, e.g., alcaine, opthaine.

Fever *chapter 21*

OBJECTIVES

After completing this chapter, you will be able to:

1. Identify normal variations in body temperature.

2. Describe two situations that should receive an emergent priority.

COMPLAINT

- Baby or child with fever or temperature
- Adult with fever or temperature
- Feels hot
- Fever and chills
- Chemotherapy patient with fever
- Cancer patient with fever
- AIDS patient with fever

> **Key Concept**
> **Signs and symptoms of fever vary tremendously.**
> **Some individuals may be asymptomatic.**

SUBJECTIVE ASSESSMENT
Present Event

- Characteristics of fever
- Temperature range
- Onset of fever

> **Key Concept**
> **Normal body temperature is lower in the morning and**
> **higher in the late afternoon. Fever generally**
> **follows the same pattern.**

- Time, drug, and dose of last antipyretic
- Effect of medication
- Associated symptoms
- Nausea, vomiting, diarrhea
- Headache
- Earache

- Respiratory symptoms

- Aching all over

- Urinary symptoms

- Back pain

- Red, swollen extremities

- Red, draining wounds

- Rash or petechiae

- Pediatric symptoms
  -Rash or petechiae

- Seizure

- Fluid intake

- Behavioral changes

Key Concept
High fever in a child can lead to febrile seizure.

History

- Chronic health problems—diabetes, malaria, spinal cord injury, hyperthyroidism

- Acute health problems—AIDS, cancer, chemotherapy, radiation, other conditions that cause immune suppression

- Exposure to potentially infectious individuals

- Toxic exposure or overdose of salicylates, phenothiazines, and others

- Recent travel to undeveloped countries

- Specific medications (e.g., antipyretics, amphetamines, tricyclic antidepressants, phenothiazines)

Key Concept
Aspirin in large quantities causes fever.
Determine amount taken.

OBJECTIVE ASSESSMENT

- Skin color, temperature, and turgor

- Oral or rectal temperature

- Mucous membrane moisture

- Work of breathing

- Orthostatic vital signs

DIAGNOSTIC PROCEDURES

- None specific for fever

INTERVENTIONS

- Remove excessive clothing

- Administer antipyretic—acetaminophen or ibuprofen

Key Concept
Never give aspirin to anyone younger than 18 years of age.

TRIAGE

Emergent

- Fever in infant younger than 3 months old

- Fever in immune-suppressed patient

- Respiratory distress

- Petechiae

Urgent

- Active vomiting

- Alert infant with reported seizure associated with fever

- Decreased fluid intake with poor skin turgor or dry mucous membranes

- High fever

Nonurgent

- Low fever and mild associated symptoms

References

Jordan, K. (Ed.). (2000). <u>Emergency nursing core curriculum</u> (5th ed.). Philadelphia: Saunders.

Kidd, P., & Sturt, P. (1996). <u>Mosby's emergency nursing reference</u>. St. Louis: Mosby.

Kitt, S., Selfridge-Thomas, J., Proehl, J., & Kaiser, J. (1995). <u>Emergency nursing: A physiologic and clinical perspective</u> (2nd ed.). Philadelphia: Saunders.

Newberry, L. (Ed.). (1998). <u>Sheehy's emergency nursing: Principles and practice</u> (4th ed.). St. Louis: Mosby.

Proehl, J. (1999). <u>Emergency nursing procedures</u> (2nd ed.). Philadelphia: Saunders.

Rosen, P., & Barkin, R. (1998). <u>Emergency medicine: Concepts and clinical practice</u> (4th ed.). St. Louis: Mosby.

Rosen, P., & Barkin, R., Hayden, S. Shaider, J. & Wolfe, R. (1999). <u>The 5 minute emergency medicine consult</u>. Philadelphia: Lippincott Williams & Wilkins.

Learning Assessment Exercises

1. A 17 year old student presents to the fever. The patient does not have a thermometer but states she has felt hot for four days. Other complaints include aching all over. Temperature is 101.4 °F, pulse 108, respirations 20, and blood pressure 112/68. Skin is warm, dry, and has a natural color. What is the most appropriate acuity for this patient?
   a. Emergent
   b. Urgent
   c. Non-urgent

2. Which of the following findings in association with high fever in an adult is cause for the greatest alarm?
   a. Vomiting
   b. Urinary frequency
   c. Aching all over
   d. Petechaie

3. Which of the following patients should receive an Emergent Priority?
   a. 6 week old with fever 102.6 °F (rectal)
   b. 88 year old with fever 100.2 °F (oral)
   c. 17 year old with temperature 103. 6 °F (oral)
   d. 55 year old with temperature 101.8 °F (oral)

4. An elderly woman comes to the ED with fever, chills, and aching all over. The patient's temperature is 104.7 °F orally. Select the patient's historical information that is most significant.
   a. Had second round of cytoxan and adriamycin a week ago.
   b. Allergic to sulfa and codeine
   c. Had a hysterectomy 10 months ago.
   d. Takes Pepcid for acid reflux.

1. Review the fever protocol used by your facility. Determine the location of antipyretic agents.

2. Discuss management of patients who may be infectious, e.g., meningitis, measles.

3. Review the procedure for management of patients who are immune suppressed.

OBJECTIVES

After completing this chapter, you will be able to:

1. Describe three complaints that should receive an emergent priority.

2. Identify three presenting symptoms indicative of stroke.

3. Discuss assessment of fluid draining from the nose or ears.

COMPLAINT

- Headache
- Head pounding
- Fainted
- Dizzy
- Unable to maintain balance
- Face hurts
- Face feels numb
- Stroke
- Loss of muscle tone or feeling on one side
- Talking funny
- One side of face is drooping
- Can't close eye
- Can't move arm or leg
- Bumped head
- Cut on head, scalp
- Scrape on head
- Laceration

SUBJECTIVE ASSESSMENT—HEADACHE

Presenting Event

- Onset of symptoms—chronic, recurrent, or acute
- Characteristics of headache
- Unilateral or bilateral, tight band around head, pulsatile in nature
- Constant, intermittent, escalating, worst headache ever experienced, only headache ever experienced
- Awakened patient from sound sleep, occurs more in evening
- Associated symptoms
- Nausea or vomiting
- Photophobia
- Dizziness or vertigo
- Visual disturbances
- Eye pain
- Fever and/or rash
- Change in memory or thinking
- Motor or sensory changes

- Stiff neck

- Ear pain

- Stuffy nose or nasal discharge

- Muscle aches or pain

- Anxiety, depression

- Prodrome of event
  -Flashing lights, funny feelings

- Time of last meal

- Caffeine consumption

- Recent head trauma—See Chapter 36: Trauma for discussion of head trauma

Key Concept
Do not ignore a patient who complains of having "the worst headache I have ever had in my life."

History

- Previous headaches like this one

- Family history of headache

- Headache history

- Type of headaches—migraine, cluster, sinus, other

- Medications that have worked

- Diagnostic tests done

- Pre-existing disease

- Hypertension

- Stroke or transient ischemic attack

- Hydrocephalus or ventricular shunt

- Environmental allergies

- Seizure

- Cancer

- Aneurysm

- Recent change in medications

- Recent change in glasses or contact lenses

- Insomnia

- Recent lumbar puncture or epidural

- Last menstrual period

- Menopausal symptoms—hot flashes, insomnia

- Specific medications (e.g., aspirin, caffeine, oral contraceptives, sedatives, narcotic analgesics, anticoagulants, anticonvulsants, antihistamines, decongestants, recreational drugs)

SUBJECTIVE ASSESSMENT—FAINTED, DIZZY, VERTIGO

Present Event

- Onset of symptoms—chronic or acute, duration of episode
- Description of the event—room spinning, sensation of movement
- Associated symptoms
- Numbness in fingers or around mouth
- Anxiety or depression
- Double vision
- Loss of hearing or ringing in ears
- Loss of coordination
- Palpitations
- Nausea or vomiting
- Loss of strength or sensation
- Duration of loss of consciousness
- Precipitating event or associated activity
  -Pain, fear, anxiety
  -Micturition
  -Defecation
  -Coughing, breath-holding episodes, or hyperventilating
  -Exertion
  -Change in position
  -Standing suddenly after eating
- Excessive food or alcohol ingestion
- Recreational drug use
- Lack of food or fluids—time of last meal or fluids
- Hot environment
- Motion sickness
- Prodrome—present or absent
- Warmth, flushing
  -Contributing conditions
- Nausea, vomiting
- Light-headedness
- Weakness

- Pallor

- Sweating

- Sensations prior to the event

- Palpitations

- Visual disturbances

- Headache

- Characteristics of recovery—alert, confused, lethargic

History
- Previous fainting episodes

- Pre-existing disease
  -Seizures
  -Diabetes
  -Hypoglycemia
  -Cardiac disease or dysrhythmias
  -Hypertension
  -Stroke or transient ischemic attack
  -Inner ear infection
  -Meniè're's disease

- Specific medications (e.g., anticoagulants, antihypertensives, cardiac medications, recreational drugs)

SUBJECTIVE ASSESSMENT—FACIAL PAIN OR UNILATERAL FACIAL PARALYSIS
Present Event
- Onset/duration of symptoms

- Description of pain—associated with jaw movement or yawning

- Swelling or discoloration

- Associated symptoms—speech impairment, visual disturbances, taste disturbances

- Head injury or blow to face

- Unilateral weakness or changes in sensation to other parts of body (see Subjective Assessment—Unilateral Weakness later in this chapter)

Key Concept
Damage to the fifth cranial nerve causes facial pain or unilateral paralysis.

History

- Previous episodes of similar pain or paralysis

- Pre-existing conditions
  -Trigeminal neuralgia
  -Bell's palsy
  -Dental abscess

- Recent facial piercings

Key Concept
Early recognition of stroke is critical. Intraveneous throm-bolytic therapy for ischemic stroke must be initiated within 3 hours of symptom onset.

SUBJECTIVE ASSESSMENT—UNILATERAL WEAKNESS, DIFFICULTY SPEAKING OR UNDERSTANDING SPEECH, OR ATAXIA

Present event

- Progression of symptoms

- Onset of symptoms—exact time is critical
  -Gradual or sudden changes

- Change in level of consciousness

- Headache, neck pain, back pain

- Motor or sensory deficits

- Speech deficits

- Taste abnormalities

- Visual disturbances

History

- Previous stroke or transient ischemic attack

- Risk factors for stroke
  -Cigarette smoking
  -Hypertension
  -Diabetes
  -Heart disease

- Other medical conditions—seizures, aneurysm, cancer, syphilis, Parkinson's disease

- Recreational drug use (e.g., amphetamines, others)

- Specific medications (e.g., anticoagulants, antihypertensive, oral hypoglycemics, insulin, cardiac medications, antiarrhythmic agents, oral contraceptives, seizure medications)

OBJECTIVE ASSESSMENT

- Neurologic assessment as appropriate
- Level of consciousness
- Patient's general state
- Infant—fussy, irritable, high-pitched cry
- Sudden behavioral changes
- Jitteriness, twitching, seizure behavior
- Glasgow Coma Scale (see Table 22-1)
- Unilateral differences in motor or sensation
- Pupil check and eye movements
- Observe for cranial nerve deficits
- Inspect and palpate head for bumps, bruises, or bleeding
- Drainage of fluid from ears or nose
- Facial asymmetry—drooping smile or ptosis
- Nuchal rigidity
- Petechiae
- Unusual odors on patient's breath
  -Alcohol
  -Fruity smell—suggests ketosis and acidosis
  -Musty odor—occurs with hepatic coma
  -Uriniferous odor—found in uremia

Key Concept
Check grip strength by matching your dominant hand to the patient's dominant hand. Eliminate pain by placing your middle finger over your index finger, and then have the patient squeeze your fingers rather than your entire hand, or your fingers placed side by side.

Table 22-1. Glasgow Coma Scale

Component	Patient	Score
Eye	Spontaneous	4
	Responds to voice	3
	Responds to pain	2
	No response	1
Verbal	Oriented	5
	Confused	4
	Inappropriate	3
	Does not make sense	2
	No verbal response	1
Motor	Obeys	6
	Localizes to stimulation	5
	Withdraws from stimulation	4
	Flexion	3
	Extension	2
	No motor activity	1

DIAGNOSTIC PROCEDURES

- Fingerstick/serum glucose

- Glucose test of fluid draining from nose or ears

- Cervical spine/skull series

- Computerized axial tomography (CT) scan

INTERVENTIONS

- Place in quiet treatment area if severe headache

- Place in dimly lit room if severe photophobia

TRIAGE

Emergent

- Possible stroke

- Headache with severe pain

- Headache followed by decreased level of consciousness

- Impaired ABCs

- Unilateral weakness—onset within 6 hours of arrival

- Sudden onset headache following exertion, coughing, or sexual activity

- Seizure activity at present

- Possible bacterial meningitis

- Ventricular shunt with history of headache or signs of infection

- First time with headache like this
- Headache with acute vision changes
- Migraine headache
- Nausea and vomiting

Nonurgent

- Sinus pain
- Toothache or temporomandibular pain

References

Jordan, K. (Ed.). (2000). <u>Emergency nursing core curriculum</u> (5th ed.). Philadelphia: Saunders.

Kidd, P., & Sturt, P. (1996). <u>Mosby's emergency nursing reference</u>. St. Louis: Mosby.

Kitt, S., Selfridge-Thomas, J., Proehl, J., & Kaiser, J. (1995). <u>Emergency nursing: A physiologic and clinical perspective</u> (2nd ed.). Philadelphia: Saunders.

Newberry, L. (Ed.). (1998). <u>Sheehy's emergency nursing: Principles and practice</u> (4th ed.). St. Louis: Mosby.

Proehl, J. (1999). <u>Emergency nursing procedures</u> (2nd ed.). Philadelphia: Saunders.

Rosen, P., & Barkin, R. (1998). <u>Emergency medicine: Concepts and clinical practice</u> (4th ed.). St. Louis: Mosby.

Rosen, P., & Barkin, R., Hayden, S. Shaider, J. & Wolfe, R. (1999). <u>The 5 minute emergency medicine consult</u>. Philadelphia: Lippincott Williams & Wilkins.

Wasson, J. (1997). <u>The common symptom guide</u> (4th ed.). New York: McGraw-Hill.

1. Which of the following patients should receive an Emergent Priority?
    a. Blood pressure 200/100 in patient with a history of hypertension
    b. Pulse of 116 in a patient with a migraine headache.
    c. Sudden onset left sided weakness in patient with atrial fibrillation
    d. History of febrile seizures in a patient with fever 100.4 °F

2. Historical information related to a complaint of headache includes:
    a. Asthma controlled by inhalers
    b. Ventricular shunt since birth
    c. New glasses 6 months ago
    d. Chronic low back pain

3. A patient with a history of migraine headaches tells you he saw flashing lights just before the pain began. The most likely explanation for this is:
    a. The flashing lights mean this headache is not a migraine headache.
    b. The flashing lights are a prodrome to a migraine headache.
    c. The flashing lights suggests a change from migraine to cluster type headaches.
    d. The flashing lights are coincidental and not related to the headache.

4. A patient with a history of hypertension presents to the ED with severe headache. The patient describes the pain as the worst headache he has ever had in his life. Which statement best describes this situation?
    a. The patient is exaggerating to get pain medicine.
    b. The patient's vital signs should be taken before an acuity determination can be made.
    c. The patient's history of hypertension is not pertinent to the complaint of headache.
    d. The patient should receive an emergency priority.

5. A 29 year old female presents to the ED with severe headache. History includes an epidural for low back pain 12 hours ago. Which of the following statements is most appropriate for this situation?
    a. The patient's age in combination with the epidural is the likely cause of her headache.
    b. There is no correlation between the headache and the epidural.
    c. The headache may be due to pressure changes caused by the epidural.
    d. The headache is a common side effect of medications injected during the epidural.

6. Determine the appropriate acuity rating for the following patients.

Acuity	Patient
————	39 year old female with headache, nausea, vomiting, and photophobia. History of migraine headaches.
————	49 year old male with severe headache, slurred speech, and difficulty walking.
————	67 year old homeless man with gum and right face pain for several days. He is alert, oriented, and ambulates normally. Speech is clear. Gums are swollen with some pus noted around several teeth.
————	10 year old female with fever, headache, and stiff neck. There are small, pinpoint spots on the chest and abdomen.
————	33 year old male with facial pressure for several days. The patient says he also has drainage running down the back of his throat. Vital signs are within normal limits. The patient is awake, alert, and oriented.

1. Review guidelines and documentation tools for neurologic assessment in your facility.

2. Identify the location of assessment tools such as pen lights and pupil charts.

Heat-Related Emergencies   *chapter 23*

OBJECTIVES

After completing this chapter, you will be able to:

1. Describe three medical conditions that place the patient at risk for a heat-related emergency.

2. Identify three conditions that should receive an emergent priority.

COMPLAINT

- Feet swollen from the heat
- Muscle cramps
- Fainted from the heat
- Too hot, can't cool down
- Sun stroke
- Overcome by heat

- Hives
- Prickly heat
- Heat rash
- Sun poisoning
- Heat stroke

> **Key Concept**
> Sodium and water loss secondary to physical activity causes muscle cramps. Treat with water and sodium replacement.

SUBJECTIVE ASSESSMENT

Present Event

- Progression of symptoms
- Activity and duration—work, recreation, other
- Environmental factors
  -Heat and humidity
  -Closed work area—tunnel, garage, silo, others
  -Occlusive clothing—bulletproof vest, fire-fighting equipment, multiple layers
  -Lack of air conditioning
- Fluid intake
- Minimal or no urine output
- Nausea and vomiting
- Headache, dizziness, weakness, and syncope
- Alcohol and recreational drug consumption
- Rash or areas of irritation

History

- Usual level of physical activity

- Age factors—pediatric or geriatric

- Medical conditions that may predispose to decreased thermoregulation
  - Alcoholism
  - Parkinsonism
  - Diabetes
  - Spinal cord injury
  - Hyperthyroidism
  - Pheochromocytoma
  - Status epilepticus
  - Pseudomotor dysfunction
  - Extensive prior burn
  - Prior heat stroke
  - Cystic fibrosis
  - Ichthyosis
  - Scleroderma
  - Ectodermal dysplasia
  - Malaria
  - Cardiovascular disease

Key Concept
The very young and the very old are at greater risk for heat-related problems because of immature or degenerating thermoregulatory mechanisms.

- Specific medications that may predispose to decreased thermoregulation
  - Anticholinergic drugs
  - Phenothiazines
  - Tricyclic antidepressants
  - Monoamine oxidase inhibitors
  - Fat-soluble sedatives or hypnotics
  - Lithium
  - Diuretics
  - Amphetamines
  - Lysergic acid diethylamide (LSD)
  - Phencyclidine
  - Cocaine
  - Beta-blockers
  - Sympatholytic antihypertensives

OBJECTIVE ASSESSMENT

- Skin color, temperature, and presence of perspiration
- Is clothing wet with sweat or dry from body heat?
- Level of consciousness
- Orientation level
- Vital signs, including temperature
- Dark urine

Key Concept
Patients with severe hyperthermia usually present with hot, dry skin; however, sweating can persist in some cases.

DIAGNOSTIC PROCEDURES

- None recommended

INTERVENTIONS

- Elevate edematous extremities
- Remove restrictive clothing

TRIAGE

Emergent

- Altered mental status
- Absence of perspiration
- Temperature $\geq$ 102 degrees F
- Elevated fever and dark urine

Urgent

- Temperature 100 to 102 degrees F
- Heat cramps

Nonurgent

- Temperature $\leq$ 100 degrees F
- Heat-related edema in lower extremities

References

Jordan, K. (Ed.). (2000). <u>Emergency nursing core curriculum</u> (5th ed.). Philadelphia: Saunders.

Kidd, P., & Sturt, P. (1996). <u>Mosby's emergency nursing reference</u>. St. Louis: Mosby.

Kitt, S., Selfridge-Thomas, J., Proehl, J., & Kaiser, J. (1995). <u>Emergency nursing: A physiologic and clinical perspective</u> (2nd ed.). Philadelphia: Saunders.

Newberry, L. (Ed.). (1998). <u>Sheehy's emergency nursing: Principles and practice</u> (4th ed.). St. Louis: Mosby.

Rosen, P., & Barkin, R. (1998). <u>Emergency medicine: Concepts and clinical practice</u> (4th ed.). St. Louis: Mosby.

Rosen, P., & Barkin, R., Hayden, S. Shaider, J. & Wolfe, R. (1999). <u>The 5 minute emergency medicine consult</u>. Philadelphia: Lippincott Williams & Wilkins.

1. The very young are at risk for heat-related emergencies because:
   a. Infants have a greater circulating blood volume.
   b. Infants do not have a mature thermoregulatory mechanism.
   c. Infants have bigger heads proportionately than adults.
   d. Infants still have a thymus gland.

2. Alcohol increases the risk for heat-related illness because the alcohol:
   a. Causes massive vasoconstriction.
   b. Increases fluid losses.
   c. Depresses the thirst mechanism.
   d. Causes sodium retention.

3. The most appropriate acuity category for the patient with heat cramps is:
   a. Emergent
   b. Urgent
   c. Non-urgent

4. A 17 year old is brought to the ED from football practice. The coach states the patient fainted during a full dress workout. The patient is pale and complains of feeling very weak. Skin is hot, but moist. Which of the following statements does NOT apply to this patient?
   a. Moist skin rules out the possibility of a heat-related emergency.
   b. Full dress workout with football gear increases the likelihood of a heat-related emergency.
   c. Fainting may be due to a heat-related emergency.
   d. Weakness is caused by fluid losses and the heat related emergency.

1. Discuss procedures for cooling the patient in the triage area.

2. Review applicable protocols for management of heat related emergencies.

Mouth *chapter 24*

OBJECTIVES

After completing this chapter, you will be able to:

1. Describe preparation of an avulsed tooth for possible reimplantation.

2. Identify two situations prioritized as emergent.

COMPLAINT

- Toothache
- Gum pain
- Bleeding from mouth or gums
- Sores in mouth
- Excessive drooling
- Funny taste in mouth
- Swelling inside mouth

- Filling fell out
- Pain after dental work
- Foreign body in cheek or tongue
- Bit tongue or cheek
- Broken or missing teeth
- Blow to jaw
- Swollen jaw

SUBJECTIVE ASSESSMENT

Present Event

- Recent dental work or oral surgery
- Trauma
- Do teeth fit together correctly when biting down?
- Can patient fully open mouth?
- Wounds to lips or inside cheeks

> **Key Concept**
> **Suspect a fractured mandible when teeth do not fit together correctly.**

History

- Dentures
  -partial, full-set
- Tongue or cheek pierced
- Cancer and/or chemotherapy
- Bleeding disorders
- Herpes simplex
- Tetanus immunization status
- Specific medications (e.g., anticoagulants, antibiotics, inhaled steroids)

OBJECTIVE ASSESSMENT

- Respiratory status
  - Is the airway open?
  - Does the voice sound normal?
  - Foreign object
    - Description and location
    - Potential for airway obstruction
- Wounds and lesions
  - Description—shape, character, open, draining
  - Location—cheek, gum, tongue, soft palate, hard palate
  - Bleeding—amount, location
  - Drainage—color, amount, location, odor
- Gum disease and general oral hygiene
  - Dental caries
  - Tooth fractures

DIAGNOSTIC PROCEDURES

- None recommended

INTERVENTIONS

- Place avulsed tooth in saline or tooth-saving solution
- Have patient bite on gauze if bleeding from extracted tooth socket
- Stabilize foreign object

TRIAGE

Emergent

- Partial or complete airway obstruction
- Uncontrolled hemorrhage
- Salvageable avulsed tooth
- Swollen tongue with airway compromise
- Severe pain
- Foreign object causing airway compromise

Urgent

- Bleeding controlled with pressure
- Foreign object through cheek into mouth without airway compromise

- Sores in mouth

- Chronic or mild tooth pain

- Swollen jaw

- Possible jaw fracture with orbital complications

References

Jordan, K. (Ed.). (2000). <u>Emergency nursing core curriculum</u> (5th ed.). Philadelphia: Saunders.

Kidd, P., & Sturt, P. (1996). <u>Mosby's emergency nursing reference</u>. St. Louis: Mosby.

Kitt, S., Selfridge-Thomas, J., Proehl, J., & Kaiser, J. (1995). <u>Emergency nursing: A physiologic and clinical perspective</u> (2nd ed.). Philadelphia: Saunders.

Newberry, L. (Ed.). (1998). <u>Sheehy's emergency nursing: Principles and practice</u> (4th ed.). St. Louis: Mosby.

Proehl, J. (1999). <u>Emergency nursing procedures</u> (2nd ed.). Philadelphia: Saunders.

Rosen, P., & Barkin, R. (1998). <u>Emergency medicine: Concepts and clinical practice</u> (4th ed.). St. Louis: Mosby.

Rosen, P., & Barkin, R., Hayden, S. Shaider, J. & Wolfe, R. (1999). <u>The 5 minute emergency medicine consult</u>. Philadelphia: Lippincott Williams & Wilkins.

1. A 33 year old male presents to triage with metal spike in the left cheek. The most appropriate first action for the triage nurse is:
   a. Identify the mechanism of injury.
   b. Assess breath sounds
   c. Stabilize the metal spike.
   d. Establish airway patency.

2. A patient involved in a motor vehicle collision complains of jaw pain. Further assessment reveals that the patient's teeth do not fit together normally. The most likely explanation for this is:
   a. Tongue dysplasia
   b. Injury to the trigeminal nerve
   c. Mandible fracture
   d. Facial edema

3. Determine the appropriate acuity for the following patients

Acuity	Description
_______	37 year old presents to the ED after being involved in a brawl. She is holding two teeth wrapped in tissue paper.
_______	14 year old tripped and bit his tongue. He has a small, horizontal laceration on front half of the tongue.
_______	49 year old with minor toothache
_______	25 year old with tongue pain and moderate drooling. Patient had tongue pierced three days ago.
_______	11 year old with severe bleeding from gums after minor dental procedure. History of hemophilia.

1. Review the procedure for management of avulsed tooth in your facility. Identify the location of the tooth-saving solution container or alternative container if not available.

2. Discuss management of false teeth–containers and the procedure for loss prevention.

OBJECTIVES

After completing this chapter, you will be able to:

1. Identify three medical problems that place the patient at risk for an emergent neck condition.

2. Describe three parameters that should be assessed on the patient with a neck complaint.

COMPLAINT

- Neck pain
- Stiff neck
- Neck twisted to one side
- Neck swollen
- Swollen glands
- Knot on neck
- Lump on neck
- Complete or partial paralysis
- Cut in neck
- Neck injury
- Neck wound
- Hit in neck
- Object stuck in neck
- Hit from behind with neck pain
- Numbness or tingling

SUBJECTIVE ASSESSMENT

Present Event

- Chronic problem or new complaint
- Onset of symptoms—gradual or sudden
- Problem unilateral or bilateral
- Progression of symptoms
- Fever and pain with flexion
- Sore throat, drooling, or difficulty swallowing
- Trauma—Refer to Chapter 36: Trauma for discussion of neck and spine trauma

> **Key Concept**
> **Fever and neck pain with flexion suggest meningitis.**

History

- Previous episodes of similar symptoms
- Exposure to meningitis
- Neck surgeries
- Vigorous exercise regimen

- New exercise program

- Recent chiropractic therapy

- Tetanus immunization status

- Hyperthyroidism

- Neck radiation

- Mononeucleosis

- Specific medications (e.g., phenothiazines [haldol, inapsine, compazine, mellaril, thorazine, reglan], muscle relaxants or analgesics)

> **Key Concept**
> **Implement appropriate isolation precautions when meningitis is suspected.**

OBJECTIVE ASSESSMENT

- Upper airway sounds such as stridor

- Subcutaneous emphysema—suggests tracheolaryngeal tear

- Hemoptysis—occurs in tracheolaryngeal tear

- Bleeding

> **Key Concept**
> **Bleeding with an expanding hematoma in the neck can compromise the airway.**

- Hoarseness or change in voice—suggests vocal cord edema or injury

- Unequal breath sounds—suggests pneumothorax or hemothorax

- Bruising or abrasions—present in tracheolaryngeal trauma or laryngeal fracture

- Laceration or puncture wound

- Motor or sensory deficits—Refer to Chapter 36: Trauma for discussion of assessment for spinal cord injury

- Range of motion for neck–if no history of injury

> **Key Concept**
> **Do not move the patient's neck when there is a history of trauma.**

- Mass in neck
  -Painful
  -Affects swallowing
  -Pulsation present

- Impaled objects
  -Bleeding around the object
  -Object moves with inspiration or pulse

DIAGNOSTIC PROCEDURES

- Cervical spine x-ray

- Soft tissue x-ray for airway obstruction

INTERVENTIONS

- Direct pressure to control bleeding and prevent air embolus
  -Use digital pressure to control carotid artery bleeding

- Stabilize foreign bodies

- Ensure cervical spine immobilization

- Ensure tetanus prophylaxis if wound present

TRIAGE

Emergent

- Partial or complete airway obstruction

- Uncontrolled bleeding

- Impaled foreign body

- Possible meningitis, epiglottitis, or retropharyngeal abscess

- Possible dystonic reaction crisis

- Acute onset hoarseness following injury

Urgent

- Neck wound with bleeding controlled, not involving deep structures

- Minor neck pain in patient in spinal immobilization

Nonurgent

- Chronic neck pain because of arthritis or previous injury with no changes in sensation or motion

- Minor neck abrasions

- Neck stiffness with no signs of infection

References

Jordan, K. (Ed.). (2000). <u>Emergency nursing core curriculum</u> (5th ed.). Philadelphia: Saunders.

Kidd, P., & Sturt, P. (1996). <u>Mosby's emergency nursing reference</u>. St. Louis: Mosby.

Kitt, S., Selfridge-Thomas, J., Proehl, J., & Kaiser, J. (1995). <u>Emergency nursing: A physiologic and clinical perspective</u> (2nd ed.). Philadelphia: Saunders.

Newberry, L. (Ed.). (1998). <u>Sheehy's emergency nursing: Principles and practice</u> (4th ed.). St. Louis: Mosby.

Rosen, P., & Barkin, R. (1998). <u>Emergency medicine: Concepts and clinical practice</u> (4th ed.). St. Louis: Mosby.

Rosen, P., & Barkin, R., Hayden, S. Shaider, J. & Wolfe, R. (1999). <u>The 5 minute emergency medicine consult</u>. Philadelphia: Lippincott Williams & Wilkins.

1. Pertinent historical information for the patient who presents with sudden onset neck pain and drooling includes:
   a. Tongue pierced 4 years ago.
   b. Took compazine 90 minutes prior to arrival.
   c. Diagnosed with mononeucleosis last week.
   d. Taking over-the-counter anti-inflammatory agents

2. Select the most appropriate triage action for a 28 year old patient who presents to the triage area with swollen glands in the neck, temperature 102. 4° F. Other vital signs are within normal limits and the patient is awake and alert.
   a. Transport immediately to the treatment area.
   b. Give an antipyretic agent.
   c. Obtain a soft tissue x-ray of the neck.
   d. Evaluate orthostatic vital signs.

3. A 15 year old patient is brought to the ED complaining of numbness and tingling of his hands and feet. The patient is slightly diaphoretic on his face, arms, and neck. The problem started during a high school wrestling match. The triage nurse should suspect what type of problem?
   a. Hyperthermia due to physical activity.
   b. Spinal cord injury
   c. Hyperventilation
   d. Excitement

4. A 42 year old patient presents to the ED with high fever and severe drooling. Which of the following statements applies to this situation?
   a. Epiglottitis is a pediatric problem so this cannot be the patient's problem.
   b. High fever suggests a viral cause for the patient's probable epiglottitis.
   c. The first priority for this patient is airway management.
   d. The most appropriate priority for this patient is urgent.

5. Determine the appropriate priority for the following patients.

Priority	Patient
_________	55 year old male with chronic neck pain who rates his discomfort as 4 on a scale of 1 to 10. No acute changes are reported.
_________	5 year old female with stiff neck and high fever. There is a pinpoint rash on face, arms, and torso.
_________	17 year old male hit in the posterior neck with baseball bat. He is awake, alert, and oriented. There is a large bruise on the neck. He moves his arms and legs on command.
_________	29 year old female with large mass on the left neck. The patient cannot swallow and has a temperature is 103. 9 F.
_________	39 year old male presents with a stiff neck. The patient states the problem started when he turned his head to the left side. The patient moves all extremities without difficulty.

1. Review protocol for epiglottitis if applicable for your facility.

2. Discuss management of the patient with possible meningitis. Determine the shortest route from triage to an isolation room or appropriate private room.

3. Identify the location for gloves and bandages for application of direct pressure. Confirm use of digital pressure when appropriate.

4. Review the procedure for spinal immobilization. Determine the time frame when this is applied to motor vehicle collision patients (up to 12 hours after the injury, up to 24 hours after the injury, etc.)

Nose *chapter 26*

OBJECTIVES

After completing this chapter, you will be able to:

1. Describe the most effective position for the patient with epistaxis.

2. Identify two complaints that should receive an emergent priority.

COMPLAINT

- Nosebleed
- Runny or stuffy nose
- Foul odor from nose
- Pus coming from nostril

- Hit in nose
- Foreign body in nose
- Nasal trauma
- Blow to nose

> **Key Concept**
> Airway clearance, blood pressure, and estimated blood loss
> are priorities for patient assessment.

SUBJECTIVE ASSESSMENT
Present Event

- Onset of symptoms—sudden or acute
- Complaint unilateral or bilateral
- Progression of symptoms
- Fever
- Sneezing
- Upper respiratory tract infection
- Color of nasal drainage
- Circumstances surrounding the event
- Duration of bleeding and estimated blood loss
- Blood running down throat

> **Key Concept**
> Epistaxis with blood running down throat
> may cause vomiting.

- Identification of object in nose
- Known injury
- Associated loss of consciousness or neck pain

History

- Previous episodes of epistaxis
- Hemophilia or other bleeding disorder
- Sinusitis
- Nasal fracture
- Environmental allergies
- Hypertension
- Headache
- Recent nasal surgery
- Recreational drug use (e.g., cocaine, inhalants, others)
- Smoker
- Tetanus immunization status
- Specific medications (e.g., anticoagulants, systemic and topical decongestants)

OBJECTIVE ASSESSMENT

- Bleeding from nostril—amount and nostril (s) involved
- Visible foreign body
- Drainage—color and consistency
- Foul odor from nose
- Swelling, ecchymosis, or deformity
- Abrasions or lacerations

DIAGNOSTIC PROCEDURES

- X-ray nasal bones if indicated

INTERVENTIONS

- Use ice pack if trauma
- Pinch nostrils together for 15 minutes to control bleeding
- Lean forward to spit out blood running down throat
- Provide tetanus prophylaxis if wound present

TRIAGE

Emergent

- Airway compromised
- Uncontrolled hemorrhage
- Epistaxis with hypertension

- Epistaxis that is partially controlled or a slow bleed
- Foreign body likely to swell

- Nasal drainage with mild discomfort
- Foreign body with mild discomfort
- Epistaxis with no bleeding at present
- Blow to nose without associated bleeding

References

Jordan, K. (Ed.). (2000). <u>Emergency nursing core curriculum</u> (5th ed.). Philadelphia: Saunders.

Kidd, P., & Sturt, P. (1996). <u>Mosby's emergency nursing reference</u>. St. Louis: Mosby.

Kitt, S., Selfridge-Thomas, J., Proehl, J., & Kaiser, J. (1995). <u>Emergency nursing: A physiologic and clinical perspective</u> (2nd ed.). Philadelphia: Saunders.

Newberry, L. (Ed.). (1998). <u>Sheehy's emergency nursing: Principles and practice</u> (4th ed.). St. Louis: Mosby.

Rosen, P., & Barkin, R. (1998). <u>Emergency medicine: Concepts and clinical practice</u> (4th ed.). St. Louis: Mosby.

Rosen, P., & Barkin, R., Hayden, S. Shaider, J. & Wolfe, R. (1999). <u>The 5 minute emergency medicine consult</u>. Philadelphia: Lippincott Williams & Wilkins.

1. Priority assessment for the patient with nose-related complaints includes:
   a. Cranial nerve evaluation
   b. Ability to speak
   c. Visual exam of the affected nostril
   d. Time of symptom onset

2. A patient presents to the triage area with a nosebleed. The triage nurse instructs the patient to lean forward during the assessment. The most appropriate explanation for this is:
   a. Leaning forward prevents blood from running down the patient's throat and causing nausea.
   b. Leaning forward allows the triage nurse to easily evaluate the amount and location of the bleeding.
   c. Leaning forward helps calm the patient by decreasing intrathoracic pressure and therefore slowing the heart rate.
   d. Leaning forward keeps old blood from contaminating the site of injury and decreases complications.

3. A 3 year old toddler is brought to the ED when the parents note a foul odor coming from the child's nose. Possible causes the triage nurse should suspect include:
   a. Septal hematoma
   b. Child abuse
   c. Severe viral infection
   d. Foreign body

4. A 24 year old male complains of nasal drying with occasional nosebleeds. Assessment shows a possible septal perforation. Pertinent historical information includes:
   a. Maxilla fracture two weeks prior to admission
   b. Frequent cocaine use
   c. Diet controlled diabetes mellitus
   d. Oral surgery last week

1. Discuss management of severe epistaxis in the triage area.

OBJECTIVES

After completing this chapter, you will be able to:

1. Identify two obstetrical complaints that require immediate attention.

2. Describe two interventions for an obstetrical emergency.

COMPLAINT

- Bleeding
- In labor
- Water broke
- Baby is coming
- Baby is not moving
- Swelling

- Cord hanging out
- Abdominal pain
- Miscarriage
- Vomiting
- Faint when I stand up
- Had a seizure

Refer to Chapter 36: Trauma for discussion of triage of the injured obstetrical patient

SUBJECTIVE ASSESSMENT
Present Event

- Description of symptoms
- Onset and duration
- Obstetrical history—grava, para, abortion, ectopic
- Last normal menstrual period
- Positive pregnancy test
  -Urine or serum
  -Home pregnancy test
- Expected date of confinement (EDC)
- Number of fetuses—single or multiple
- Abdominal pain or pelvic pain
  -Quality, severity, characteristics, timing, and provocation
- Nausea and vomiting
- Fever or chills
- Vaginal bleeding or discharge
  -Amount, color, quality, and odor
  -Itching or burning

- Membranes ruptured
  -When and associated color and odor
- Fetal movement
  -No movement or change in movement
- Urinary symptoms
  -Frequency, burning, urgency, hematuria, pressure
- Visual disturbances
- Headache
- Sudden weight gain
- Dependent or generalized edema
- Shoulder pain

Key Concept
Assess rapidly to determine if delivery is imminent. Know the location of the precipitous delivery tray for your facility.

History

- Reproductive history
- Number of pregnancies, abortions (spontaneous and therapeutic), deliveries, and living children
- Prenatal care if appropriate
- Date and type of delivery if postpartum
- History of obstetrical complications
- History of ectopic pregnancy
- Contraceptive use
- Blood type and Rh factor if known
- Sexual history—new partner in past 2 months or multiple partners in past 6 months
- Medical history
- Cardiac disease
- Abdominal and/or pelvic surgery
- Pulmonary disease
- Diabetes
- Thyroid disease
- Renal disease
- Hypertension
- Sexually transmitted disease (STD)
- Substance abuse—tobacco, alcohol, recreational drugs
  -Time and amount of last consumption

- Specific medications (e.g., pain medications, antiemetics, prenatal vitamins, others)

OBJECTIVE ASSESSMENT

- Orthostatic blood pressure and pulse
- Level of consciousness
- Skin color, temperature, and moisture
- Edema—facial, peripheral, or generalized
- Vaginal bleeding/fluids
  -Color, odor, and amount
  -Presence of amniotic fluid
  -Presence of clots or tissue
  -Presence of meconium
- Fetal assessment
  -Fetal heart tones if greater than 12 weeks gestation
  -Fetal activity
- Uterine contractions—pattern, duration, and intensity

DIAGNOSTIC PROCEDURES

- Serum glucose if altered level of consciousness or history of diabetes

INTERVENTIONS

- Support airway, breathing, and circulation
- Position in left lateral recumbent position if greater than 20 weeks gestation
- Determine current seizure activity
- Support on side, if possible, to promote drainage of oral secretions
- Loosen tight or restrictive clothing
- Protect the abdomen, limbs, and head from injury

TRIAGE

Emergent

- Crowning
- Impending delivery
- Vaginal hemorrhage
- Ruptured membranes
- Severe abdominal pain
- Labor pains less than 15 minutes apart
- Significant change in orthostatic vital signs
- Seizure activity or reported seizure

- Altered level of consciousness
- Severe hypertension
- Fetal heart tones less than 120 or greater than 160

- Labor pains more than 15 minutes apart
- Vaginal discharge or urinary symptoms with fever
- Vaginal bleeding with normal vital signs and normal fetal heart tones

Nonurgent

- Vaginal discharge without fever or associated symptoms

References

Jordan, K. (Ed.). (2000). <u>Emergency nursing core curriculum</u> (5th ed.). Philadelphia: Saunders.

Kidd, P., & Sturt, P. (1996). <u>Mosby's emergency nursing reference</u>. St. Louis: Mosby.

Kitt, S., Selfridge-Thomas, J., Proehl, J., & Kaiser, J. (1995). <u>Emergency nursing: A physiologic and clinical perspective</u> (2nd ed.). Philadelphia: Saunders.

Newberry, L. (Ed.). (1998). <u>Sheehy's emergency nursing: Principles and practice</u> (4th ed.). St. Louis: Mosby.

Rosen, P., & Barkin, R. (1998). <u>Emergency medicine: Concepts and clinical practice</u> (4th ed.). St. Louis: Mosby.

Rosen, P., & Barkin, R., Hayden, S. Shaider, J. & Wolfe, R. (1999). <u>The 5 minute emergency medicine consult</u>. Philadelphia: Lippincott Williams & Wilkins.

1. A 17 year old pregnant patient (12 weeks gestation) presents to the ED with severe vaginal bleeding. The triage nurse should:
   a. Take the patient to the labor and delivery area.
   b. Position the patient on the left side.
   c. Transport the patient to the nearest treatment area.
   d. Perform a digital exam to rule out prolapsed cord.

2. A patient who is 33 weeks pregnant presents with pains 7 to 8 minutes apart. Rapid visual assessment reveals a prolapsed umbilical cord. The most appropriate action for the triage nurse is:
   a. Raise the patient's head 30 to 45 degrees.
   b. Use a gloved hand to lift the vaginal wall off the cord.
   c. Ask the patient to push.
   d. Wait five minutes and reassess.

3. A patient who is 36 weeks gestation presents to the ED with confusion, elevated blood pressure, and severe edema. The most appropriate priority for this patient is:
   a. Emergent
   b. Urgent
   c. Non-urgent

4. You have a patient who is full term with severe back pain. She states her water broke 4 hours ago. You place the patient on a stretcher for transport to labor and delivery. What other action should you take before transport?
   a. Place the patient on the right side.
   b. Loosen the patient's pants.
   c. Raise the patient's head.
   d. Insert an intravenous catheter.

1. Identify the location of the precipitous delivery tray.

2. Determine the shortest route from the triage area to the nearest room for emergent delivery.

3. Determine the shortest route from the triage area to the labor and delivery area.

4. Review the procedure for management of the patient with a prolapsed cord.

Psychiatric Complaint *chapter 28*

OBJECTIVES

After completing this chapter, you will be able to:

1. Describe three characteristics of a psychiatric emergency.

2. Identify two psychiatric complaints that require immediate attention.

COMPLAINT

- Can't stop crying
- Depressed
- Hearing voices
- Want to die
- Want to kill self
- Want to commit suicide
- Psychotic
- Freaking out
- Flipped out
- Lost it

- Anxiety attack
- Panic attack
- Bizarre behavior
- "Crazy"
- Violent behavior toward self or others
- Cutting, stabbing, or hitting self
- Hitting, cutting, stabbing others
- Flashbacks
- Screaming, shrieking uncontrollably
- Decompensated

SUBJECTIVE ASSESSMENT

Present Event

- Reason for coming to the ED from the patient
- Reason for coming to the ED from those with the patient

> **Key Concept**
> The patient may not know why he or she has been brought to the ED. Obtain information from the patient and anyone with the patient.

- Alcohol use in past 24 hours
    - Time of last drink
- Drug use in past 24 hours
    - Type and route of use
    - Time of last consumption
- Physical complaints
- Suicidal
    - Does the patient have a plan?
    - Does the patient have means to carry out the plan?

•Paranoid
   -"Someone is out to get me or hurt me."

- Visual, auditory, and/or tactile hallucinations
- Individual(s) with patient
   -Supportive and cooperative
   -Intoxicated
   -Potentially violent
   -Cooperative
   -Victim of domestic violence

History

- Psychiatric history
- Diagnoses
   -Panic disorders, bipolar disorder, phobias, anxiety disorder, conversion disorder, hyperventilation syndrome, post traumatic stress disorder, others
- Treatment
- Hospitalizations
- Previous suicide attempts
   -Number of attempts
   -Method of attempts
- Previous episodes of violence
   -Violence directed at self
   -Violence directed at others
- Recreational drug use
- Alcohol abuse
- Family and social history
   -Domestic violence
   -Child abuse
   -Homeless
- Family history of schizophrenia
- Medical conditions—acute and chronic

- Home situation—homeless, previously institutionalized

- Specific medications (e.g., psychotropic drugs, anticholinergic drugs)

Key Concept
Medical conditions that disrupt cerebral function or cause metabolic abnormalities can exacerbate psychiatric pathology.

OBJECTIVE ASSESSMENT

- Potential for violence

- Cooperative or uncooperative

- Verbal communication
  - Bizarre word use
  - Grandiose ideas
  - Flight of ideas
  - Rapid but fluent expression of ideas
  - Sexual content in every conversation
  - Disjointed, garbled, difficult to understand
  - Repeats everything that is said

- Affect
  - Flat or catatonic
  - Euphoric or elation
  - Flamboyant or impulsive

- Current behavior
  - Repetitive motions or behaviors
  - Level of orientation
  - Eye contact

- Hygiene
  - Clothing—dirty, tattered, multiple layers, bizarre combinations
  - Person—dirty hair and body, odors, possible infestations

- Belongings
  - No personal belongings with patient
  - All belongings with patient

- Injuries—new, old, or various states of healing

- Rashes

- Nutritional state

DIAGNOSTIC PROCEDURES

- Serum alcohol
- Drug levels for substance(s) of abuse
- Fingerstick glucose/serum glucose
- Breath alcohol level
- Serum electrolytes

INTERVENTIONS

- Intervene for potential violence
- Restrain if immediate threat to self or others
- Remove potential weapons—knives, cigarette lighters, pills, needles
- Call support person(s)

TRIAGE

Emergent

- Immediate danger to self or others
- Possible toxic ingestion

Urgent

- High suicide potential
  -May be emergent if unaccompanied
- High risk for leaving before treatment
  -May be emergent if unaccompanied

Nonurgent

- Chronic condition and requesting medication refill
- Low suicide risk and cooperative

References

Drury, T. (1999). How to defuse a walking time bomb. <u>Nursing Management, 30</u>(3), 59-61.

Glasson, L. (1993). Preparation, staff awareness, preventive practices, and the psychiatric patient. <u>Journal of Emergency Nursing, 19</u>(5), 385-391.

Hoag-Apel, C. (1998). Violence in the ED. <u>Nursing Management, 29</u>(7), 60-63.

Hoag-Apel, C. (1999). Smart safeguards for the ED: Preventing rising ED violence from striking your unit. <u>Nursing Management, 30</u>(5), 31-33.

Jordan, K. (Ed.). (2000). <u>Emergency nursing core curriculum</u> (5th ed.). Philadelphia: Saunders.

Kidd, P., & Sturt, P. (1996). <u>Mosby's emergency nursing reference</u>. St. Louis: Mosby.

Kitt, S., Selfridge-Thomas, J., Proehl, J., & Kaiser, J. (1995). <u>Emergency nursing: A physiologic and clinical perspective</u> (2nd ed.). Philadelphia: Saunders.

Nield-Anderson, L., & Doubrava, J. (1993). Defusing verbal abuse: A program for ED triage nurses. <u>Journal of Emergency Nursing, 19</u>(5), 441-445.

Newberry, L. (Ed.). (1998). <u>Sheehy's emergency nursing: Principles and practice</u> (4th ed.). St. Louis: Mosby.

Point of View. (1998, August). Violence in the workplace. <u>Point of View Magazine</u>, pp. 4-6.

Rosen, P., & Barkin, R. (1998). <u>Emergency medicine: Concepts and clinical practice</u> (4th ed.). St. Louis: Mosby.

Rosen, P., & Barkin, R., Hayden, S. Shaider, J. & Wolfe, R. (1999). <u>The 5 minute emergency medicine consult</u>. Philadelphia: Lippincott Williams & Wilkins.

Williams, M., & Roberston, K. (1997). Workplace violence: Prevalence, prevention, and first-line interventions. <u>Critical Care Nursing Clinics of North America, 9</u>(2), 221-228.

1. A 47 year old male with history of alcohol abuse presents to the ED with severe hallucinations. The patient is agitated and extremely diaphoretic. Vital signs are temperature 102.6 degrees F, pulse 136, respirations 32, and blood pressure 170/120. What is the most critical historical information for this patient.
   a. Smokes 2 packs of cigarettes per day.
   b. Last drink 2 days prior to admission.
   c. Lives with his mother who is also an alcoholic
   d. Works at a local chemical plant.

2. A patient who presents to the ED after attempting to harm himself should be:
   a. Searched for potential weapons.
   b. Placed in four point restraints
   c. Left alone until police arrive
   d. Removed to the police holding cell.

3. An elderly woman is brought by her family because she is not acting like herself. The family states she has a history of hypertension, diabetes, and coronary artery disease. She has been recently depressed after the death of her sister. The most appropriate initial diagnostic procedure for this patient is:
   a. Breath alcohol test
   b. Fingerstick glucose
   c. Electrocardiogram
   d. CT scan of the head

4. What is the appropriate priority for the following patients?

   Acuity   **Patient**

   _______   17 year old male who is hearing voices for several days. This usually happens when he doesn't take his medicine. Vital signs are within normal limits. The patient does not remember the last time he took his medicine.

   _______   29 year old female found wandering on the street by the police. The patient does not know who she is or where her family is. Her clothing is torn and covered with blood splatters.

43 year old female is brought to the ED for treatment of drug abuse. The patient is agitated and refuses help. She has used cocaine in increasing amounts for the past five days. Family is with her.

____

26 year old male is brought to the ED by his wife. She is very concerned because he will not stop washing his hands. He tells you he doesn't know what is wrong, but he just needs to wash his hands. Problem has gradually worsened over the past month.

____

59 year old male arrives by EMS. He smells of alcohol. He is awake and yelling, his clothing is covered with vomit. EMS personnel report the patient was found on his lawn after his wife locked him out of the house.

____

A 9 year old male is brought to the ED by his parents after he repeatedly cut his arms and legs with broken pieces of glass.

1. Identify the location of emergency 'panic' buttons in the triage area. Review the procedure for getting help if a patient becomes violent in triage.

2. Review the management of the suicidal patient in your facility. Discuss applicable protocols for these patients.

OBJECTIVES

After completing this chapter, you will be able to:

1. Identify two objective parameters for triage of the patient with a respiratory complaint.

2. Describe two respiratory complaints that require immediate attention.

COMPLAINT

- Can't breathe
- Trouble breathing
- Rattling in chest
- Hurts to breathe
- Wheezing
- Choking
- Hoarse
- Fever and chills
- Chest hurts
- Back hurts
- Cold
- Flu
- Croup
- Breathing too fast

- Hyperventilating
- Coughing
- Spitting up blood
- Coughing up blood
- Night sweats
- Turning blue
- Tuberculosis (TB)
- Overcome by smoke
- Inhaled something poisonous
- Pneumonia
- Emphysema
- Lung problem
- Lung trouble
- Fluid in chest

> **Key Concept**
> Respiratory distress causes great anxiety and
> fear for most people. Reassure the patient
> while you assess the complaint.

SUBJECTIVE ASSESSMENT
Present Event
- Description of problem
- Onset of symptoms
  -Duration and pattern of symptoms—acute or chronic
  -Worse at night
  -How many pillows do you sleep on?

- Precipitating event
  -None
  -Coughed or took a deep breath
  -Breathed fumes, smoke, or other form of chemical
  -Got something stuck in throat or windpipe
  -Exercise
  -Got upset or emotional
  -Diving
  -Mountain climbing

- Fever and/or chills

- Night sweats

- Audible wheezing or rattling in chest

- Pain in chest or back
  -Hurts to breathe
  -Hurts on one side
  -Radiating or nonradiating

- Cough
  -Wheezing, barking, or dry cough
  -Productive or nonproductive
  -Worse at night
  -Color and thickness of sputum
  -Blood in sputum

- Hoarseness

- Associated neck swelling

- Ache all over

- Edema
  -Legs or entire body

- Sweating, pale, dizziness

- Gets better with rest or change in position

- Calf or leg pain

- Rash or hives

- Refer to Chapter 15: Chest for triage of the patient with a chest complaint.

- Refer to Chapter 34: Throat for triage of the patient with a throat complaint.

- Refer to Chapter 35: Toxicities for triage of the patient exposed to smoke or other toxic fumes.

- Refer to Chapter 36: Trauma for triage of the patient with chest trauma.

History

- Pulmonary disease
  - Recent respiratory infection
  - Emphysema, chronic obstructive pulmonary disease (COPD), asthma, bronchitis, pneumocystis

- Cardiac disease
  - Congestive heart failure (CHF)
  - Cardiomyopathy
  - Atrial fibrillation or atrial flutter
  - Heart transplant

- Renal disease
  - Dialysis patient

- Autoimmune disorders
  - HIV/AIDS

- Chemotherapy or radiation therapy
  - Cancer patient
  - Lung cancer
  - Metastatic disease

- Exposure to known allergen
  - Environmental
  - Medication
  - Food

- Drug overdose
  - Heroin

- Multisystem insult

- Shock
  - Postoperative
  - Postpartum

- Obesity

- Social history

- Cigarette smoker
  - Duration and amount per day
  - Pipe or cigarette
  - Filtered or unfiltered

- Ethanol use

- Occupational hazards—firefighter, coal miner, cotton mill worker, chemical plant worker, silo worker

- Recreational drug use
  -Marijuana, inhalants, heroin, cocaine, amphetamines
  -Intravenous drug use

- Prolonged sitting or travel

- Recent travel to mountainous region

- Alternative therapy—home remedies, health food or herbs

- Specific medications (e.g., anticoagulants, cardiac medications, antibiotics, anti-hypertensives, oral hypoglycemics, insulin, antacids, analgesics, home oxygen, nebulizer treatments)

OBJECTIVE ASSESSMENT

- Respiratory rate, rhythm, and depth

- Respiratory effort
  -Obvious exertion
  -Use of accessory muscles
  -Nasal flaring
  -Intercostal and/or substernal retractions
  -Bulging intercostal spaces

- Oxygen saturation level

- Blood pressure and pulse

- Pulsus paradoxus

- Skin color, temperature, and moisture

- Circumoral cyanosis

- Dusky or cyanotic nailbeds

- Capillary refill time

- Mucosal color, temperature, and moisture

- Level of consciousness
  -Restless, anxious, confused

- Breath sounds
  -Present or absent
  -Increased or decreased
  -Distribution through lung fields
  -Abnormal breath sounds
  -Audible to the ear
  -Wheezing or musical sounds
  -Crackles or rales

- Friction rub

- Posture or position of comfort

- Carpopedal spasms

- Tingling around mouth or in hands and feet

- Neck vein distention

- Tracheal deviation

- Edema
    -Peripheral, central

- Pitting—amount

> **Key Concept**
> More than 25 different rales are described in most medical dictionaries. If you do not know which sound the patient is making, it is better to describe what you hear rather than attempt to label it.

DIAGNOSTIC TESTS

- Chest x-ray

- Electrocardiogram

- Peak expiratory flow rate

INTERVENTIONS

- Support airway, breathing, and circulation

- Administer oxygen

- Transport by wheelchair to decrease oxygen demand

- Position for effective air movement

- Apply appropriate mask if tuberculosis is known or suspected

TRIAGE

Emergent

- Respiratory distress

- Oxygen saturation less than 90 percent

- Altered level of consciousness with respiratory compromise

- Suspected croup or epiglottitis

- Patient unable to speak because of respiratory distress

- Audible wheezes after exposure to a known allergen

- Frothy pink secretions with respiratory compromise

- Shortness of breath with normal pulse oximetry reading

- Cough with fever, history of lung or heart disease, or elderly patient

- Asthma patient with pulsus paradoxus greater than 20 mm Hg

- Hyperventilation with carpopedal spasms

- Cough without fever or respiratory compromise

- Mild upper respiratory infection

ESI 5-Level Model

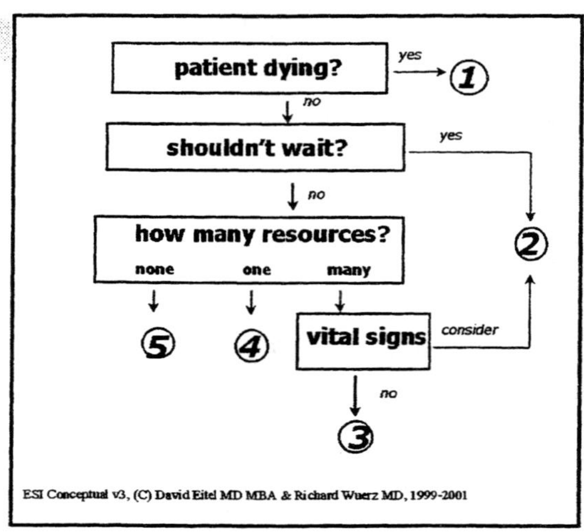

References

Jordan, K. (Ed.). (2000). <u>Emergency nursing core curriculum</u> (5th ed.). Philadelphia: Saunders.

Kidd, P., & Sturt, P. (1996). <u>Mosby's emergency nursing reference</u>. St. Louis: Mosby.

Kitt, S., Selfridge-Thomas, J., Proehl, J., & Kaiser, J. (1995). <u>Emergency nursing: A physiologic and clinical perspective</u> (2nd ed.). Philadelphia: Saunders.

Newberry, L. (Ed.). (1998). <u>Sheehy's emergency nursing: Principles and practice</u> (4th ed.). St. Louis: Mosby.

Rosen, P., & Barkin, R. (1998). <u>Emergency medicine: Concepts and clinical practice</u> (4th ed.). St. Louis: Mosby.

Rosen, P., & Barkin, R., Hayden, S. Shaider, J. & Wolfe, R. (1999). <u>The 5 minute emergency medicine consult</u>. Philadelphia: Lippincott Williams & Wilkins.

1. The patient with severe respiratory distress also has frothy pink secretions. The most likely explanation for this is:
   a. Chemical contamination
   b. Pulmonary edema
   c. Medication for pneumonia
   d. Unresolved pulmonary infection

2. Which of the following statements applies to the patient who is taking medication for tuberculosis?
   a. The patient is still contagious since you do not know the type of tuberculosis he has.
   b. The patient is still contagious because the medication regimen is not completed.
   c. The patient is still contagious until three negative AFB smears are obtained.
   d. The patient is still contagious but does not require complete respiratory isolation.

3. A patient presents to the ED complaining of a dry scratchy throat and cough for a week. The patient has a history of hypertension and thyroid problems. What historical data can add to the clinical assessment of this patient?
   a. Date of last thyroid profile
   b. Started new blood pressure medicine ten days ago.
   c. Works as comptroller for a local airline.
   d. Takes multivitamins with iron each day.

4. A 19 year old female presents to the ED with severe spasms of both hands. She is very pale, diaphoretic, and has a respiratory rate of 48 per minute. The most likely explanation for this situation is:
   a. Carpopedal spasms due to hyperventilation
   b. Allergic reaction caused by latex allergy
   c. Hypercalcemia secondary to overdose
   d. Carpal tunnel syndrome with severe pain

5. Determine the appropriate triage acuity for the following patients.

Acuity	Patient
_______	79 year old male with severe dyspnea worsening over the past 12 hours. The patient tells you he has to sleep in his recliner. There is severe pitting edema to mid calf.
_______	17 year old female with expiratory wheezing after eating shrimp. The patient's lips are swollen and edematous.
_______	29 year old female who is coughing. The patient also complains of aching all over and mild to moderate fever.
_______	48 year old male with frothy pink secretions and severe respiratory distress. Family reports the patient became sick after shooting up heroin.
_______	33 year old female complains of trouble breathing. Oxygen saturation and vital signs are within normal limits. The patient states the problem has gotten worse over the past 2 days.
_______	68 year old female with moderate respiratory distress. Respirations are 36 per minute and shallow. Moderate pedal edema is noted. There are fine crackles heard over both sides of the chest.

6. Determine the appropriate ESI 5-Level catagories for the above patients.

1. Walk the path from triage to the appropriate treatment areas for patient with severe respiratory distress.

2. Describe assessment for the patient with potential tuberculosis. Identify the location for masks and guidelines for application. Determine the location of the negative airflow room in your facility.

3. Review management of severe anaphylaxis in the triage area.

Seizure *chapter 30*

OBJECTIVES

After completing this chapter, you will be able to:

1. Identify two emergent complaints related to seizure.

2. Name two diagnostic procedures for the patient with a seizure.

COMPLAINT

- Seizure
- Had a fit
- Fell down and shook
- Epilepsy
- Shaking on one side of body or one part of body
- Fainted
- Fell out
- Tingling or numbness
- Problem with vision, hearing, smell, or taste
- Shaking all over

> **Key Concept**
> **Grand mal seizure is usually followed by a postictal period characterized by confusion and memory loss.**

SUBJECTIVE ASSESSMENT
Present Event

- Time of seizure
- Description of seizure activity
  - Motor activity
  - Loss of consciousness
  - Shaking
  - Body part(s) involved
  - Respiratory status during seizure
  - Duration and frequency of seizure
  - Incontinence
  - Ocular deviation
  - Sensory problems—vision, taste, smell, or hearing
  - Numbness or tingling

> **Key Concept**
> **Ask anyone with the patient to describe the seizure.**

- Patient status after seizure
  - Level of consciousness, orientation
  - Injuries because of seizure activity

- Associated aura
  - -Foul smell
  - -Metallic or bitter taste
  - -Flashing lights
  - -Buzzing, ringing, or hissing sounds
- Preceding events
  - -Blow to head
  - -Fainted
  - -Holding breath
  - -Headache
  - -Fever

History

- Epilepsy
- Alcohol abuse
  - -History of seizures secondary to withdrawal
  - -Time of last drink
  - -Usual alcohol consumption

Key Concept
Seizures related to alcohol withdrawal can occur 12 to 24 hours after the patient's last drink.

- Drug abuse
  - -Substance(s) used
  - -Route used—inhaled, oral, intravenous, other
  - -Time of last consumption
  - -History of seizures secondary to ingestion or withdrawal
- Previous brain injury or surgery
- Cancer—type and presence of metastatic disease
- HIV status
- Hypertension
- Cerebral aneurysm
- History of febrile seizure in infant or child
- Diabetes
- Specific medications (e.g., anticonvulsant, antihypertensive, insulin or other anti-hyperglycemic agents)

Key Concept
Seizures can occur when a patient's medication has been changed or when other medications alter effects of the anticonvulsant.

OBJECTIVE ASSESSMENT

- Current tonic-clonic seizure activity
- Respiratory effectiveness
- Body parts involved
- Ocular deviation
- Progression of seizure activity
- Duration of seizure
- Number of seizures and length of each episode
- Distinct episodes with recovery between each seizure
- Status epilepticus
- Level of consciousness
- Ability to follow commands
- Response to stimuli
- Presence of automatism
- Level of orientation
- Headache
- Amnesia
- Associated weakness in one limb
- Presence of rash or purpura
- Associated injuries

DIAGNOSTIC PROCEDURES

- Serum level of prescribed anticonvulsants
- Serum ethanol
- Serum level of other drugs
- Fingerstick/serum glucose
- Breath alcohol level

INTERVENTIONS

- Manage current seizure activity
- Support on side, if possible, to promote drainage of oral secretions
- Loosen tight or restrictive clothing
- Protect limbs and head from injury

TRIAGE

Emergent

- Current generalized seizure activity
- Decreased level of consciousness or confusion
- Fever with seizure
- Compromised airway
- No history of seizures
- Recent head trauma

Urgent

- Focal seizure activity with history of same
- No history of seizures, no seizure activity now, alert and oriented

Nonurgent

- History of seizures, no seizure activity now, alert and oriented
- Patient ran out of medicine and feels as though a seizure might happen

References

Cline, D.M., & Ma, O.J. (1996). *Emergency medicine: A comprehensive study guide* (4th ed.). New York: McGraw-Hill.

Jordan, K. (Ed.). (2000). *Emergency nursing core curriculum* (5th ed.). Philadelphia: Saunders.

Kidd, P., & Sturt, P. (1996). *Mosby's emergency nursing reference*. St. Louis: Mosby.

Kitt, S., Selfridge-Thomas, J., Proehl, J., & Kaiser, J. (1995). *Emergency nursing: A physiologic and clinical perspective* (2nd ed.). Philadelphia: Saunders.

Newberry, L. (Ed.). (1998). *Sheehy's emergency nursing: Principles and practice* (4th ed.). St. Louis: Mosby.

Proehl, J. (1999). *Emergency nursing procedures* (2nd ed.). Philadelphia: Saunders.

Rosen, P., & Barkin, R. (1998). *Emergency medicine: Concepts and clinical practice* (4th ed.). St. Louis: Mosby.

Rosen, P., & Barkin, R., Hayden, S. Shaider, J. & Wolfe, R. (1999). *The 5 minute emergency medicine consult*. Philadelphia: Lippincott Williams & Wilkins.

Wasson, J. (1997). *The common symptom guide* (4th ed.). New York: McGraw-Hill.

1. A patient presents to the ED complaining of a metallic taste in his mouth. He says there is a buzzing in his ears and he cannot think straight. His current medications are tegretol and multivitamins. The most likely cause of this problem is:
    a. Hallucinations secondary to vitamin toxicity.
    b. The patient is drunk or high on drugs.
    c. The patient may have psychomotor seizures.
    d. The patient has taken a drug overdose.

2. Confusion and amnesia following an epileptic seizure is called the:
    a. Post ictal period
    b. Post prandial period
    c. Post seizure period
    d. Post coital period

3. The first priority for the patient who has a seizure in the triage area is:
    a. Transport the patient immediately to the treatment area.
    b. Protect the patient from curious onlookers
    c. Place the patient on the side to prevent aspiration.
    d. Obtain IV access

4. Determine the appropriate priority for the following patients.

Acuity	Patient
_______	17 year old patient who had a seizure two hours before arrival. The patient has not taken his seizure medicine for two days. He is awake, alert, and vital signs are within normal limits.
_______	58 year old patient with a history of alcohol abuse. The patient's last drink was yesterday. The patient arrives by ambulance. He is awake but confused. His tongue is oozing a small amount of blood.
_______	33 year old patient comes to the ED with twitching of his left arm. He sees a doctor for this problem.

1. Discuss management of the seizure patient in the triage area.

Sexual Assault *chapter 31*

OBJECTIVES

After completing this chapter, you will be able to:

1. Identify two situations related to sexual assault that require immediate attention.

2. Describe three subjective parameters essential to triage of the victim of sexual assault.

COMPLAINT

- Raped
- Assaulted
- Sodomized
- Hurt
- Molested

Key Concept

Sexual assault is not gender-specific—the victim may be female or male. Information required for triage of any victim of sexual assault is the same regardless of gender.

SUBJECTIVE ASSESSMENT

Present Event

- Date, time, and place of the assault
- Description of the assault
  - Attempted or completed
  - Vaginal, oral, rectal penetration
  - Foreign objects used
  - Condom used
  - Number of assailants
  - Force used
- Associated injuries
- Post-assault activities
  - Bathed or showered
  - Douche, enema
  - Brushed teeth, gargled
  - Urination, defecation
  - Changed clothing
- No memory of the event

History

- Last normal menstrual period
- Contraceptive use
- Consenting intercourse within 72 hours of attack
- Reproductive history
- Recent gynecologic treatment or surgery
- History of sexually transmitted diseases (STD) or pelvic inflammatory disease
- Tetanus immunization status
- Substance abuse—alcohol or other recreational drugs
- Current medications (e.g., contraceptives, others)

OBJECTIVE ASSESSMENT

- Emotional status and behavior
- Condition of clothing, nails, and skin (e.g., dirty, torn, stained)
- Obvious injuries—bite marks, bruises, lacerations, others

DIAGNOSTIC TESTS

- None indicated for triage

INTERVENTIONS

- Provide psychosocial support for patient
- Preserve clothing and other items for evidence
- Instruct the patient not to urinate, wash the perineum, or gargle until the examination is completed

TRIAGE

Emergent

- Sexual assault with altered level of consciousness or abnormal vital signs

- Severe emotional distress

Urgent

- Sexual assault with no obvious emotional distress, no changes in level of consciousness, and normal vital signs

Nonurgent

- Sexual assault more than 24 hours prior to arrival with no emotional or physical distress

References

Emergency Nurses Association (ENA). (2000). *Emergency nursing core curriculum* (5th ed.). Philadelphia: Saunders.

Kidd, P., & Sturt, P. (1996). *Mosby's emergency nursing reference*. St. Louis: Mosby.

Kitt, S., Selfridge-Thomas, J., Proehl, J., & Kaiser, J. (1995). *Emergency nursing: A physiologic and clinical perspective* (2nd ed.). Philadelphia: Saunders.

Newberry, L. (1998). *Sheehy's emergency nursing: Principles and practice* (4th ed.). St. Louis: Mosby.

Rosen, P., & Barkin, R. (1998). *Emergency medicine: Concepts and clinical practice* (4th ed.). St. Louis: Mosby.

Rosen, P., & Barkin, R., Hayden, S. Shaider, J. & Wolfe, R. (1999). *The 5 minute emergency medicine consult*. Philadelphia: Lippincott Williams & Wilkins.

1. The victim of sexual assault tells you she showered before she came to the hospital. Which of the following statements about documentation applies to this situation.
   a. This is essential data for evidence collection and analysis and should be documented.
   b. This is essential information for determining validity of the attack and should be documented.
   c. This is essential information for assessment of the patient's state of mind and should be documented.
   d. This is essential information for meeting requirements established by JCAHO and should be documented.

2. A 21 year old female comes to the ED because she thinks she was raped. She tells you she woke up with sticky substance on her legs and pubic area, but does not remember being attacked. She says she was at a party last night, but is adamant that she has never has sexual intercourse. The most likely explanation for this is:
   a. The patient is denying her first sexual encounter.
   b. The patient was given something by her attacker.
   c. The patient is hallucinating due to stress.
   d. The patient is experiencing an abnormal menstrual cycle.

3. Determine the appropriate triage acuity for the following patients.

   Acuity   **Patient**

   _______   33 year old female who states she was assaulted two days ago. She is alert and vital signs are within normal limits.

   _______   11 year old female brought by parents after she was assaulted by two teens. She is agitated and screaming uncontrollably.

   _______   29 year old male states he was attacked by two men. There is severe bleeding noted on the patient's pants leg. Blood pressure is 98/50 and pulse is 138.

   _______   29 year old female who states she was assaulted 2 hours ago. She is calm but quiet. Her vital signs are within normal limits.

1. Review applicable protocols for management of the victim of sexual assault.

2. Discuss use of the SANE if appropriate for your facility.

Skin Problems *chapter 32*

OBJECTIVES

After completing this chapter, you will be able to:

1. Identify two complaints that require immediate attention.

2. Describe two interventions for skin problems related to allergic reaction.

COMPLAINT

- Rash
- Hives
- Itching all over
- Bumps on skin
- Poison ivy
- Poison oak
- Latex allergy
- Swelling
- Redness
- Pustules
- Scalp problems
- Lice
- Scabies

SUBJECTIVE ASSESSMENT

Present Event

- Progression of symptoms—acute or chronic

> **Key Concept**
> **A patient with rapid progression of symptoms is at greater risk for respiratory involvement and possible anaphylaxis.**

- Exposure to others with similar rash or hives
- Exposure to possible allergen or irritant
- Pre-existing illness
- Systemic complaints
  -Shortness of breath
  -Fever
  -Nausea and vomiting
  -Headache
  -Weakness
  -Dizziness or near syncope
- Exposure to someone with lice or scabies

History

- Known allergens—drugs, foods, latex, others

- Previous rashes or hives

- Treatment prior to arrival
  - Medications (e.g., epinephrine, antihistamine, steroids)
  - Alternative therapy—MSG paste, tobacco paste, others

- Latex allergy

- School outbreak of lice or scabies

- HIV status

- Specific medications—any new medications or change in regimen

OBJECTIVE ASSESSMENT

- Respiratory status
  - Wheezing
  - Shortness of breath
  - Stridor

- Character of rash or hives
  - Location and extent
  - Color
  - Texture
  - Macular—flat and red
  - Papular—red and raised
  - Vesicles—bumps filled with fluid
  - Bullae—very large papules

- Firmness

- Shape or pattern
  - Bull's eye, others

- Skin characteristics away from problem area

- Color, temperature, presence of diaphoresis

- Visible infestation of lice or scabies

DIAGNOSTIC PROCEDURES

- None recommended

INTERVENTIONS

- Avoid contact with the patient's clothing, skin, or hair unless wearing gloves if the patient:

  -Was exposed to a known allergen (e.g., poison ivy, poison oak)

  -Has an obvious infestation of lice or scabies

- Separate the patient with lice or scabies from other patients and visitors

- Apply temporary dressings for lesions with severe drainage

TRIAGE

Emergent

- Respiratory distress

- Signs of impending anaphylaxis

- Purpura in febrile patient

Urgent

- Uncomplicated hives with severe itching

Nonurgent

- Uncomplicated rash

- Lice or scabies

References

Cline, D.M., & Ma, O.J. (1996). <u>Emergency medicine: A comprehensive study guide</u> (4th ed.). New York: McGraw-Hill.

Jordan, K. (Ed.). (2000). <u>Emergency nursing core curriculum</u> (5th ed.). Philadelphia: Saunders.

Kidd, P., & Sturt, P. (1996). <u>Mosby's emergency nursing reference</u>. St. Louis: Mosby.

Kitt, S., Selfridge-Thomas, J., Proehl, J., & Kaiser, J. (1995). <u>Emergency nursing: A physiologic and clinical perspective</u> (2nd ed.). Philadelphia: Saunders.

Newberry, L. (Ed.). (1998). <u>Sheehy's emergency nursing: Principles and practice</u> (4th ed.). St. Louis: Mosby.

Proehl, J. (1999). <u>Emergency nursing procedures</u> (2nd ed.). Philadelphia: Saunders.

Rosen, P., & Barkin, R. (1998). <u>Emergency medicine: Concepts and clinical practice</u> (4th ed.). St. Louis: Mosby.

Rosen, P., & Barkin, R., Hayden, S. Shaider, J. & Wolfe, R. (1999). <u>The 5 minute emergency medicine consult</u>. Philadelphia: Lippincott Williams & Wilkins.

Wasson, J. (1997). <u>The common symptom guide</u> (4th ed.). New York: McGraw-Hill.

1. A patient presents to the ED with diffuse urticaria over the face, arms, and torso. The most critical historical finding for this patient is:
   a. The patient's symptoms have gotten worse over the past hour.
   b. The patient has had previous episodes.
   c. The patient does not remember what he is allergic to.
   d. The patient has severe itching due to the urticaria.

2. The first priority for the patient with an allergic reaction is:
   a. Determine the appropriate triage priority.
   b. Identify the cause of the reaction.
   c. Assess the patient's airway.
   d. Review the patient's allergies.

3. Determine the appropriate triage acuity for the following patients.

Acuity	Patient
_______	44 year old female with severe respiratory distress after eating shrimp.
_______	19 year old male with faint rash on torso which started 5 days ago. Symptoms have not worsened over time.
_______	29 year old female with red rash around the waist and the top of her legs. No other symptoms.
_______	59 year old male with fever 104.8 F and purpura on chest and abdomen.
_______	48 year old female who says she has something crawling in her hair. She thinks she has been exposed to lice.
_______	35 year old male with hives over entire body. He is complaining of severe itching.

1. Discuss management of the patient with a communicable skin condition, e.g., chicken pox, measles, lice. Determine the most appropriate treatment area for each.

2. Discuss management of the patient with anaphylaxis in the triage area.

3. Review management of the patient with a latex allergy.

Surface Wounds *chapter 33*

OBJECTIVES

After completing this chapter, you will be able to:

1. Identify two surface wounds that require immediate attention.

2. Describe two triage interventions for surface wounds.

COMPLAINT

- Cut skin
- Scraped skin
- Bruised skin
- Puncture wound
- Bleeding from an injury
- Stepped on nail
- Abrasion
- Laceration
- Grease gun injury
- Nail gun injury
- Rug burn
- Road rash
- Need stitches

SUBJECTIVE ASSESSMENT - INJURIES
Present Event

- Time of injury
- Mechanism of injury
- Location on body
- Number of wounds
- Wound contamination
- Estimated blood loss
- Change in sensation or movement
- Color and temperature of affected area
- Refer to Chapter 13: Bites and Stings for triage of bites and stings.
- Refer to Chapter 19: Extremity for triage of extremity injuries with bone involvement.
- Refer to Chapter 36: Trauma for triage of the trauma patient.

> **Key Concept**
> Treat as a trauma patient when there has been a significant mechanism of injury.

History

- Hemophilia and other conditions that prolong bleeding
- Diabetes mellitus, steroid therapy, and other conditions that impair healing
- Tetanus immunization status
- Specific medications (e.g., anticoagulants, steroids)

OBJECTIVE ASSESSMENT

- Description of wound
- Location
- Type of wound—laceration, incision (cut), abrasion, avulsion, bruise, puncture
  -Combination of above
- Length and depth of wound
- Shape—gaping, linear, irregular border
- Tissue appearance
- Amount and character of bleeding
- Evidence of arterial involvement
- Contamination—amount and type
- Foreign body—location and type

> **Key Concept**
> **Wounds that require sutures should not wait more than
> 4 hours for evaluation.**

DIAGNOSTIC PROCEDURES

- X-rays to rule out bone injury or locate foreign body

INTERVENTIONS

- Remove constrictive clothing
- Remove rings and watches from affected limb
- Position for comfort and to control bleeding
- Apply dressing to protect wound, contain drainage, and control bleeding
- Administer tetanus prophylaxis per facility protocol
- Apply splint to prevent further injury, stabilize foreign body, and provide comfort

TRIAGE

Emergent

- Uncontrolled bleeding

- Decreased perfusion distal to injury

- Grease gun injection

> **Key Concept**
> Grease gun injection is associated with massive tissue destruction beneath the skin. Immediate debridement is required.

Urgent

- Impaired sensation or motor function

- Large, complicated, or multiple surface injury

- Bleeding disorders or anticoagulant treatment

- Orbital or facial cellulitis

- Other significant cellulitis

- Grossly contaminated wound(s)

Nonurgent

- Abrasions

- Contusions

- Minor lacerations, incisions, or puncture wounds

References

Cline, D.M., & Ma, O.J. (1996). <u>Emergency medicine: A comprehensive study guide</u> (4th ed.). New York: McGraw-Hill.

Jordan, K. (Ed.). (2000). <u>Emergency nursing core curriculum</u> (5th ed.). Philadelphia: Saunders.

Kidd, P., & Sturt, P. (1996). <u>Mosby's emergency nursing reference</u>. St. Louis: Mosby.

Kitt, S., Selfridge-Thomas, J., Proehl, J., & Kaiser, J. (1995). <u>Emergency nursing: A physiologic and clinical perspective</u> (2nd ed.). Philadelphia: Saunders.

Newberry, L. (Ed.). (1998). <u>Sheehy's emergency nursing: Principles and practice</u> (4th ed.). St. Louis: Mosby.

Proehl, J. (1999). <u>Emergency nursing procedures</u> (2nd ed.). Philadelphia: Saunders.

Rosen, P., & Barkin, R. (1998). <u>Emergency medicine: Concepts and clinical practice</u> (4th ed.). St. Louis: Mosby.

Rosen, P., & Barkin, R., Hayden, S. Shaider, J. & Wolfe, R. (1999). <u>The 5 minute emergency medicine consult</u>. Philadelphia: Lippincott Williams & Wilkins.

Wasson, J. (1997). <u>The common symptom guide</u> (4th ed.). New York: McGraw-Hill.

1. A 26 year old male presents to the ED with a laceration on his left calf. Vital signs are within normal limits. Critical historical information for this patient is:
   a. Patient came to the ED by private automobile
   b. The patient takes multivitamins every day.
   c. Walks five miles every day
   d. History of hemophilia

2. Which of the following clinical findings indicates the need to prioritize a palm laceration as emergent?
   a. The patient has never received tetanus immunization.
   b. The laceration is irregular and gaping. Bleeding is present but stops with elevation and dressing application.
   c. The patient is on anticoagulants following heart valve replacement two months ago. No bleeding or bruising is noted.
   d. The second finger is pale and cool to the touch. The patient can flex the finger but cannot extend it.

3. A 39 year old male comes to the ED with an injury to his left forearm. There is a small puncture wound with some swelling noted. Which of the following mechanisms of injury indicates this patient should be given an emergent priority?
   a. Injured by a wire thrown from a lawn mower.
   b. Injured by a nail that ricocheted from a nail gun.
   c. Injured by a grease gun in the garage where he worked.
   d. Injured by a stick when he fell while walking in the woods.

4. A 15 year old female presents to the ED with a laceration of her upper lip. Which of the following assessment findings suggests this wound requires special attention?
   a. The laceration was caused by a piece of metal.
   b. The laceration goes beyond the vermillion border.
   c. The laceration goes through to the inside of her lip.
   d. The laceration was caused by the patient's metal braces on the upper teeth.

5. Determine the appropriate priority for the following patients.

Acuity	Patient
_______	33 year old female with severe redness and swelling around her left eye.
_______	18 year old male with large laceration of the left wrist from falling through a plate glass window. The wound is jagged and there is a large amount of bright red blood spurting from the wound.
_______	78 year old female with small area of tissue pulled back on the right forearm. Patient does not remember how it happened. Neurovascular exam is normal.
_______	44 year old female with crush injury of the left upper arm. The patient has several lacerations on the upper and lower arm. The radial pulse is diminished and the patient cannot move her fingers.

1. Determine the location of dressing supplies in the triage area. Discuss protocols for cleaning wounds.

2. Review protocols for tetanus prophylaxis in triage if appropriate for your facility.

Throat *chapter 34*

OBJECTIVES

After completing this chapter, you will be able to:

1. Identify two complaints that should receive an emergent priority.

2. Discuss assessment of the patient with airway compromise secondary to obstruction.

COMPLAINT

- Sore throat
- Swollen throat
- Swollen tonsils
- Hives with throat swelling
- Cough
- Hoarse voice
- Change in voice
- Swollen glands
- Bleeding following surgery
- Swallowed caustic liquid
- Difficulty swallowing or can't swallow
- Something in throat
- Swallowed a coin
- Hit in throat

SUBJECTIVE ASSESSMENT

Present Event

- Onset of symptoms—gradual or sudden
- Complaint—unilateral or bilateral
- Respiratory difficulty
- Ability to swallow
- Exposure to an allergen
- Identification of foreign body
- Exposure to chemicals
- Exposure to smoke or super-heated air
- Trauma to neck or larynx
- Fever
- Recent tonsillectomy, adenoidectomy, or other throat surgery

History

- History of allergic reactions
- Condition that may cause obstruction (e.g., throat deformities, injury, surgery)
- Radiation to throat

OBJECTIVE ASSESSMENT

- Upper airway sounds such as stridor
- Drooling or inability to swallow saliva
- Redness, swelling, or exudate in posterior pharynx
- Swelling, bruising, or subcutaneous emphysema of anterior neck

DIAGNOSTIC PROCEDURES

- Rapid strep test
- Soft tissue x-ray for airway obstruction

INTERVENTIONS

- Keep the patient who is drooling calm. Do not insert anything into mouth. Do not have the patient lie flat.
- Allow the pediatric patient who is drooling to remain in his or her parent's arms.

TRIAGE

Emergent

- Partial or complete upper airway obstruction
- Impending anaphylaxis
- Hemorrhage
- Possible laryngeal fracture
- Possible croup or epiglottitis

Urgent

- Foreign body with no respiratory involvement

Nonurgent

- Sore throat without airway compromise
- Cough without respiratory compromise

References

Jordan, K. (Ed.). (2000). <u>Emergency nursing core curriculum</u> (5th ed.). Philadelphia: Saunders.

Kidd, P., & Sturt, P. (1996). <u>Mosby's emergency nursing reference</u>. St. Louis: Mosby.

Kitt, S., Selfridge-Thomas, J., Proehl, J., & Kaiser, J. (1995). <u>Emergency nursing: A physiologic and clinical perspective</u> (2nd ed.). Philadelphia: Saunders.

Newberry, L. (Ed.). (1998). <u>Sheehy's emergency nursing: Principles and practice</u> (4th ed.). St. Louis: Mosby.

Rosen, P., & Barkin, R. (1998). <u>Emergency medicine: Concepts and clinical practice</u> (4th ed.). St. Louis: Mosby.

Rosen, P., & Barkin, R., Hayden, S. Shaider, J. & Wolfe, R. (1999). <u>The 5 minute emergency medicine consult</u>. Philadelphia: Lippincott Williams & Wilkins.

1. A 33 year old female presents to the ED with severe hoarseness. Critical historical information includes:
   a. Taking medications for hypertension.
   b. Cleaning her bathroom with chlorine solution.
   c. No known allergies.
   d. Braces applied two months ago.

2. A 4 year old patient is brought to the ED with high fever. On exam you notice the child has severe drooling. The most appropriate action for this situation is:
   a. Remove the patient from the mother's arms and transport immediately to the treatment area.
   b. Leave the patient in the mother's arms and transport immediately to the treatment area.
   c. Obtain the child's temperature and pulse oximetry.
   d. Exam the child's posterior pharynx for the presence of a foreign body.

3. A 9 year old male is brought to the ED with severe bleeding following a tonsillectomy. The most appropriate priority for this patient is:
   a. Emergent
   b. Urgent
   c. Non-urgent

4. A 27 year old female comes to the ED after she is hit in the throat with a softball. The most significant assessment finding for this patient is:
   a. There is a small bruise on her throat.
   b. She cannot speak above a whisper.
   c. Her blood pressure is 144/68.
   d. Her temperature is normal.

1. Review location of emergent airway supplies in the triage area.

2. Discuss protocols for management of the patient with epiglottitis if applicable for your facility.

3. Discuss management of the patient experiencing anaphylaxis in the triage area.

Toxicities *chapter 35*

OBJECTIVES

After completing this chapter, you will be able to:

1. Describe two objective indicators of toxicity-related problems.

2. Identify two toxicity situations that require immediate attention.

COMPLAINT

- Took too many pills
- Overdose
- Took too much medicine
- Inhaled gasoline
- Tried to commit suicide
- Want to kill myself
- Smoke inhalation
- Take special herbs or dietary supplements
- Splashed something in eye(s)
- Someone put something in my drink
- Drank something from under the sink or chemicals in the garage

- Shot up
- Shot too much of a drug
- Injected unknown drug
- Sniffing glue
- Sniffing aerosols
- Huffing aerosols
- Smoking pot
- Smoking crack
- Smoking other substances
- Hallucinations

Refer to Chapter 20: Eye for triage of ocular contamination.

Refer to Chapter 7: Violence for discussion of violence in the ED.

Refer to Chapter 30: Seizure for triage of a patient with seizures.

SUBJECTIVE ASSESSMENT
Present Event

- Identification of substance(s)
- Time and amount of intake
- Route of exposure—oral, nasal, intravenous, rectal, or others
- Containers, vials, or pill bottles at scene
- Vomiting
  -Pill fragments
  -Frequency
  -Color
- Does not remember anything
- Level of orientation—confused, drowsy, lethargic, agitated, violent, euphoric

- Ringing in ears

- Severe sweating

- Trouble walking

- Reason for consumption
  -Consumption not confirmed, only suspected
  -Accidental
  -Recreational
  -Suicide attempt

History

- Psychiatric disorders

- Recreational drug use

- Substance(s) of choice—Table 35-1 highlights common recreational drugs

- Usual consumption, route of administration, and pattern or use

Table 35-1. Common Recreational Drugs

Type	Example	Street Name or Brand Name
Narcotics	Heroin	Horse, H, Smack, Dope, Boy, Stuff
	Morphine	MS
	Meperedine	Demerol
	Sublimaze	Fentanyl
Stimulants	Amphetamines	Crank, Ice, Meth, Speed, Crystal, Crystal Meth
	Cocaine	Coke, Crack, Snow
Hallucinogens	Phencyclidine	Angel Dust, PCP, Hog
	Lysergic Acid	LSD, Acid, Mickey Mouse, Paper Acid, Blotter Acid
Cannabis	Marijuana	Grass, Pot, Weed, THC, AcapulcoGold
Sedative-Hypnotics	Benzodiazepines	Valium, Versed
	Barbiturates	Seconal
	Nonbenzodiazepines	Buspar, Quaalude, Zolpram, Meprobamate

- Drug and/or alcohol abuse/addiction

- Usual consumption—substance, amount, and pattern of use

- Previous suicide attempts

- Occupational hazards

- Dermal hazards

- Inhalation hazards

- Social hazards
  - -Bar hopping, heavy drinking, indiscriminate partying
- Infection history
  - -Hepatitis, HIV, syphilis, tuberculosis, endocarditis
- Recent stressful events
- Alternative therapies
- Herbs or natural supplements—gingoba, gamma hydroxybutyrate (GHB), body-building supplements
- Specific medications (e.g., psychotropic agents, sedative-hypnotics, vitamins with iron, others)

> **Key Concept**
> GHB is a dietary supplement available through various nutrition and health food stores. Recreational use has increased significantly in the past 5 years, leading to an increased number of ED visits.

OBJECTIVE ASSESSMENT

- Respiratory status since intake
  - -Depressed respiratory effort
  - -Tachypnea
- Altered level of consciousness
  - -Confused
  - -Agitated, violent
  - -Comatose
  - -Loss of consciousness at scene—duration
- Seizure activity
- Ocular abnormalities
  - -Dilated and sluggish
  - -Pinpoint and non-reactive
- Nystagmus
- Unusual odors (see Table 35-2)
- Burns or residue in or around mouth
- Needle marks—new and old
- Emesis or gastric contents
  - -Pill fragments
  - -Abnormal color

<table>
<tr><td colspan="2" align="center">Table 35-2. Odors Associated with Toxicity</td></tr>
<tr><td>Odor</td><td>Substance</td></tr>
<tr><td>Almonds</td><td>Cyanide poisoning</td></tr>
<tr><td>Gasoline</td><td>Gasoline ingestion or inhalation</td></tr>
<tr><td>Ammonia</td><td>Ammonia ingestion or inhalation</td></tr>
<tr><td>Violets</td><td>Turpentine ingestion or inhalation</td></tr>
<tr><td>Garlic odor</td><td>Organophosphate poisoning</td></tr>
<tr><td>Fruity odor</td><td>Ketones secondary to salicylate toxicity</td></tr>
</table>

- Skin abnormalities
  - Rash or blisters
  - Jaundice, flushed, or other discoloration
  - Hot and dry
  - Excessive diaphoresis
- Gastric abnormalities
  - Diarrhea, vomiting, excessive salivation
- Related injuries—bruises, abrasions, lacerations, others

DIAGNOSTIC PROCEDURES

- Serum ethanol level
- Serum or urine levels for suspected or known drugs
- Breath alcohol test
- Serum glucose

> **Key Concept**
> Do not assume changes in level of consciousness are related to drug intoxication. Rule out hypoglycemia, hypoxia, and other correctable causes.

INTERVENTIONS

- Support ABCs in the patient with altered level of consciousness
- Protect the violent or agitated patient from harm
- Safeguard others in the area
- Remove potential weapons—pills, needles, other substances
- Help arrange psychiatric support if suicide attempt is suspected

TRIAGE

Emergent

- Suspected intake of toxic substances in toxic amounts
- Respiratory distress or ineffective respiratory effort
- Altered level of consciousness
- Violent or agitated patient following drug consumption
- Hallucinations in a patient with a history of violence

Urgent

- Suicide attempt with normal level of consciousness and normal vital signs
- Marijuana or alcohol consumption with minimal alterations in level of consciousness and normal vital signs

Nonurgent

- Nontoxic ingestion and stable psychiatric condition

References

Cline, D.M., & Ma, O.J. (1996). <u>Emergency medicine: A comprehensive study guide</u> (4th ed.). New York: McGraw-Hill.

Dart, R.C. (2000). <u>The 5 minute toxicology consult</u>. Philadelphia: Lippincott Williams & Wilkins.

Jordan, K. (Ed.). (2000). <u>Emergency nursing core curriculum</u> (5th ed.). Philadelphia: Saunders.

Kidd, P., & Sturt, P. (1996). <u>Mosby's emergency nursing reference</u>. St. Louis: Mosby.

Kitt, S., Selfridge-Thomas, J., Proehl, J., & Kaiser, J. (1995). <u>Emergency nursing: A physiologic and clinical perspective</u> (2nd ed.). Philadelphia: Saunders.

Newberry, L. (Ed.). (1998). <u>Sheehy's emergency nursing: Principles and practice</u> (4th ed.). St. Louis: Mosby.

Proehl, J. (1999). <u>Emergency nursing procedures</u> (2nd ed.). Philadelphia: Saunders.

Rosen, P., & Barkin, R. (1998). <u>Emergency medicine: Concepts and clinical practice</u> (4th ed.). St. Louis: Mosby.

Rosen, P., & Barkin, R., Hayden, S. Shaider, J. & Wolfe, R. (1999). <u>The 5 minute emergency medicine consult</u>. Philadelphia: Lippincott Williams & Wilkins.

Wasson, J. (1997). <u>The common symptom guide</u> (4th ed.). New York: McGraw-Hill.

1. A 48 year old patient comes to the ED after ingesting an unknown amount of aspirin. The patient is awake, but slightly confused. The face is flushed and skin is hot to the touch. The most appropriate priority for this patient is:
   a. Emergent
   b. Urgent
   c. Non-urgent

2. Which of the following statements is true about inhalant abuse?
   a. These are low toxicity agents.
   b. Inhalants cause respiratory and neurologic compromise.
   c. Use is limited to a very small area in the United States.
   d. There is only one way to abuse inhalants.

3. A very large 22 year old patient who abuses stimulants presents to the triage area. The patient is loud, sweating profusely, and very agitated. The risk for violence in triage is directly related to:
   a. Any pre-existing psychiatric conditions
   b. The stimulants.
   c. The patient's size.
   d. The triage nurse's attitude.

4. A 13 year old female comes to the ED with nausea, vomiting, and jaundice. The patient states she took a bottle of acetaminophen several days ago. The most appropriate priority for this patient is:
   a. Emergent
   b. Urgent
   c. Non-urgent

5. A 59 year old alcoholic is brought to the ED by police. They state he is 'drunk again.' The patient is stuporous but does not smell of alcohol. Vital signs are within normal limits, but you note an irregular pulse. The first diagnostic procedure for the triage nurse to perform is:
   a. Serum ethanol
   b. Fingerstick glucose
   c. CT scan of the head
   d. Electrocardiogram

1. Review toxicity problems common for your facility. Discuss street drugs frequently seen in your facility.

2. Determine the location of panic buttons for triage. Review the procedure for summoning help should a patient become violent.

3. Identify the procedure for contacting Poison Control.

OBJECTIVES

After completing this chapter, you will be able to:

1. Describe three clinical presentations that require immediate attention.

2. Define four essential components for triage of the trauma patient.

COMPLAINT

- Trauma
- Hurt
- Beat up, assaulted, hit
- Car wreck
- Motorcycle crash
- Bike crash
- Fall
- Paralyzed after fall, car crash, gunshot wound, or stabbing

- Hit by car
- Shot
- Stabbed
- Cut
- Nail gun injury
- Something impaled in body
- Boating accident
- Fell off roof, out of tree
- In an explosion

Refer to Chapter 14: Burns for triage of the patient with a burn injury.

> **Key Concept**
> **Obtain pertinent information from patient, bystanders, police, or EMS personnel.**

SUBJECTIVE ASSESSMENT—GENERAL

Present Event

- Mechanism of injury
  - Blunt
    - Motor vehicle collision
    - Motorcycle collision
    - Bicycle crash
    - Pedestrian
    - Fall
    - Assault
  - Penetrating
    - Gunshot
    - Stabbing
    - Other
- Description of the event

-Precipitating events
-How the injury occurred
-Time elapsed since injury
-Treatment prior to arrival

- Events surrounding the injury
  -Accidental
  -Intentional
  -Because of patient or another person

- Protective equipment use
  -Lap belt, shoulder harness, air bags, safety seat
  -Helmet, goggles
  -Protective clothing
  -Bulletproof vest

- Loss of consciousness or change in level of consciousness

- Difficulty breathing

- Location of injuries

- Obvious blood loss

- Severe pain

- Associated symptoms

- Nausea and/or vomiting

- Headache

- Can't move arms or legs

- Pregnant

- Alcohol or other recreational drugs involved

SUBJECTIVE ASSESSMENT—BLUNT INJURY
Present Event
Motor Vehicle Collision

- Type of motor vehicle
  -Car, truck, motorcycle, boat, other
  -Size and other pertinent characteristics

- Position at time of the collision
  -Driver or passenger
  -Location in the vehicle

- Description of collision
  -Rear end, head-on, broad-side/T-bone, rollover, rotational
  -Hit another vehicle, tree, railing, other
  -Thrown from vehicle
  -Speed at impact

- Vehicle damage
    -Steering wheel broken
    -Steering column broken
    -Passenger space intrusion from door or engine
- Extrication required
- Vehicle landed in water
- Vehicle fire
- Death in vehicle
- Restraint devices
    -Lap belt, shoulder harness, air bag
    -Safety seat
- Helmet
- Goggles
- Protective clothing

Pedestrian Injury

- Type of vehicle that caused injury
- Size and other pertinent characteristics
- Position at time of impact
- Facing vehicle
- Struck from behind
- Struck from side

Key Concept
Children tend to face forward at impact, whereas adults turn sideways so they receive lateral impact.

- Description of collision
    -Occurred on street, dirt road, or open field
    -Hit and thrown from vehicle
    -Knocked down and run over
    -Landed on hard or soft surface

Injuries from Falls

- Events preceding the fall
    -Tripped and fell
    -Diving or jumping
    -Pushed
    -Don't remember
- Description of the fall
    -Distance fallen

-Landing surface
  ▪Water—pool, river, lake, ocean
  ▪Solid surface—concrete, asphalt, wooden surface, metal
  ▪Ground—rocks, mud, clay, sand, grass
-Position at impact
  Sitting, standing, landed on head, landed on back

> **Key Concept**
> **Severity of injuries from a fall is determined by the distance fallen, landing surface, position at impact, and age of the patient.**

Assault Injuries

- Events surrounding the event
  -Sports related—football, rugby, other contact sport
  -Altercation between strangers
  -Altercation between individuals known to each other

- Weapon used
  -Fists
  -Wooden bat or other wooden object
  -Metal objects—chains, chairs, spikes
  -Other objects

SUBJECTIVE ASSESSMENT—PENETRATING INJURY

Present Event

Gunshot

- Events surrounding the injury
  -Accidental
  -Self-inflicted
  -Shot by unknown assailant
  -Shot by known assailant

- Description of weapon
  -Handgun, rifle, shotgun

- Type of ammunition—hollow point, other

- Relationship of gun to victim

- Distance from weapon to victim

- Trajectory—weapon up, down, or level with victim

- Description of wounds
  -Location and number
  -Small or large, minimal tissue damage or massive destruction
  -Powder residue present

- Other wounds noted
  -Abrasions, lacerations, burns, or bruising

Stabbing or Other Penetrating Injury

- Description of events surrounding the injury
  - Accidental
  - Self-inflicted
  - Stabbed by unknown assailant
  - Stabbed by known assailant
  - Injured by nail gun
  - Injured during a fall
    - Distance of fall
    - Type of landing surface

- Description of the weapon
  - Length, width, and shape
  - Other characteristics—metal, wood, glass

- Description of wounds
  - Wounding object still in place
  - Location and number of wounds
  - Small or large, minimal tissue damage or massive destruction

- Other wounds noted
  - Abrasions, lacerations, burns, or bruising

- Relationship of weapon to victim

- Assaulted from the front, back, or side

- Assailant much taller or much shorter than victim

History

- Trauma history—previous injuries and treatment

- Medical conditions—asthma, diabetes, heart disease, hypertension, seizure disorder

- Surgical procedures

- Obstetrical history
  - Pregnancy known—length of gestation and expected date of delivery
  - Pregnancy suspected—date of last normal menstrual period

- Tetanus immunization status

- Recreational drug use—alcohol, marijuana, cocaine, others

- Specific medications (e.g., narcotics, cardiac medications, antihypertensive medications, antiseizure medications, antidepressants, psychotropic medications)

OBJECTIVE ASSESSMENT

- Complete primary assessment (see Table 36-1)

- Complete secondary assessment if appropriate (see Table 36-2)

- Signs of drug abuse—needle tracks, contraband on patient

Table 36-1. Primary Assessment

Assessments	Interventions
A = Airway with Simultaneous Cervical Spine Stabilization and/or Immobilization	
While maintaining spinal stabilization:	•Position the patient
•Vocalization	•Jaw thrust or chin lift
•Tongue obstruction	•Suction or remove foreign objects
•Loose teeth or foreign objects	•Oro/nasopharyngeal airway
•Bleeding	•Cervical spine stabilization
•Vomitus or other secretions	•Endotracheal intubation
•Edema	•Needle or surgical cricothyrotomy
B = Breathing	
•Spontaneous breathing	•Supplemental oxygen
•Chest rise and fall	•Bag-valve-mask ventilation
•Skin color	•Needle thoracentesis
•General rate and depth of respirations	•Chest tube
•Soft tissue and bony chest wall integrity	•Nonporous dressing taped on 3 sides
•Use of accessory and/or abdominal muscles	
•Bilateral breath sounds	
•Jugular veins and position of trachea	
C = Circulation	
•Pulse general rate and quality	•Direct pressure over uncontrolled bleeding sites
•Skin color, temperature, degree of diaphoresis	•Two large-bore intravenous catheters with warmed lactated Ringer's solution or normal saline
•External bleeding	•Infuse fluid rapidly with blood tubing or trauma IV tubins
	•Blood sample for typing
	•Pericardiocentesis
	•ED thoracotomy
	•Cardiopulmonary resuscitation and advanced life support measures
	•Blood administration
	•Surgery
D = Disability (neurologic status)	
•Level of consciousness (AVPU)	•Perform further investigation
•Pupils (PERL)	•Hyperventilation, if indicated

Adapted from: Emergency Nurses Association (ENA). (2000). *Trauma nursing core curriculum* [Provider Manual] (5th ed.). Des Plaines, IL: Author. p 131-132

Table 36-2. Secondary Assessment

E = Expose Patient/Environmental Control (remove clothing and keep patient warm)

•Remove clothing

•Blankets

•Warming lights

F = Full Set of Vital Signs/Five Interventions/Facilitate Family Presence

•In addition to obtaining a complete set of vital signs

•Consider: these five interventions

  -Cardiac monitor

  -Pulse oximeter (SpO_2)

  -Urinary catheter if not contraindicated

  -Gastric tube

  -Laboratory studies

•Facilitate family presence

G = Give Comfort Measures

•Verbal reassurance

•Touch

•Pain control

H = History

History	•MIVT
	•Patient-generated information
	•Past medical history

H = Head-To-Toe Assessment

Head and face	•Inspect for wounds, ecchymosis, deformities, drainage from nose and ears, and check pupils
	•Palpate for tenderness, note bony crepitus, deformity
Neck	•Remove the anterior portion of the cervical collar to inspect and palpate the neck. Another team member must hold the patient's head while the collar is being removed and replaced.
	•Inspect for wounds, ecchymosis, deformities, and distended neck veins
	•Palpate for tenderness, note bony crepitus, deformity, subcutaneous emphysema, and tracheal position
Chest	•Inspect for breathing rate and depth, wounds, deformities, ecchymosis, use of accessory muscles, paradoxical movement
	•Auscultate breath and heart sounds
	•Palpate for tenderness, note bony crepitus, subcutaneous emphysema, and deformity
Abdomen and flanks	•Inspect for wounds, distention, ecchymosis, and scars
	•Auscultate bowel sounds
	•Palpate all four quadrants for tenderness, rigidity, guarding, masses, and femoral pulses
Pelvis and perineum	•Inspect for wounds, deformities, ecchymosis, priapism, blood at the urinary meatus or in the perineal area
	•Palpate the pelvis and assess anal sphincter tone

<table>
<tr><th colspan="2" style="text-align:center">Table 36-2. Secondary Assessment</th></tr>
<tr><td colspan="2">H = Head-To-Toe Assessment</td></tr>
<tr><td>Extremities</td><td>•Inspect for ecchymosis, movement, wounds, and deformities
•Palpate for pulses, skin temperature, sensation, tenderness, deformities, and note bony crepitus</td></tr>
<tr><td colspan="2">I = Inspect Posterior Surfaces</td></tr>
<tr><td>Posterior surface</td><td>•Maintain cervical spine stabilization and support injured extremities while the patient is logrolled
•Inspect posterior surfaces for wounds, deformities, and ecchymosis
•Palpate posterior surfaces for tenderness, and deformities
•Evaluate anal sphincter tone (if not performed previously)</td></tr>
</table>

Adapted from: Emergency Nurses Association (ENA). (2000). *Trauma nursing core curriculum* [Provider Manual] (5th ed.). Des Plaines, IL: Author. p 131-132

> **Key Concept**
> Trauma in the pregnant patient who is less than 20 weeks gestation involves only one patient. Trauma in the patient who is more than 20 weeks gestation involves two patients—the mother and the neonate.

DIAGNOSTIC PROCEDURES

- Determined by findings of primary assessment (see Table 36-1)
- Determined by findings of secondary assessment (see Table 36- 2)

INTERVENTIONS

- Determined by findings of primary assessment (see Table 36-1)
- Determined by findings of secondary assessment (see Table 36-2)

> **Key Concept**
> Never cut through powder residue, bullet holes, or holes from other weapons.

TRIAGE

Emergent

- Impaired airway, breathing, or circulation
- Decreased level of consciousness
- Hemodynamic compromise
- Profound shock
- Penetrating trauma of head, neck, chest, abdomen, pelvis, or groin

- Paralysis or priapism
- Child pedestrian
- Pregnant trauma victim
- Amputation of hand, arm, foot, or leg
- Two or more proximal long-bone fractures
- Flail chest

Urgent

- Head injury with possible loss of consciousness—now alert and oriented
- Single proximal long bone fracture with normal vital signs
- Any patient on long spine board with normal vital signs

Nonurgent

- Minor injuries in patient with normal vital signs
- Isolated fracture of hand or foot with normal vital signs and minimal pain

ESI 5-Level Model

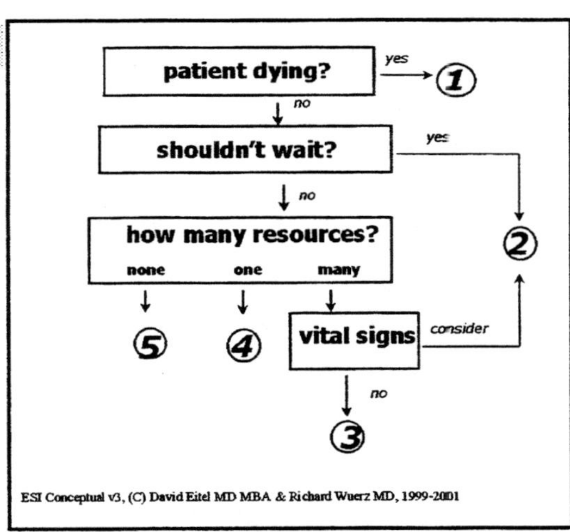

References

Emergency Nurses Association. (2000). <u>Trauma nursing core curriculum</u> [Provider Manual] (5th ed.). Des Plaines, IL: Author.

Jordan, K. (Ed.). (2000). <u>Emergency nursing core curriculum</u> (5th ed.). Philadelphia: Saunders.

Feliciano, D., Moore, E., & Mattox, K. (1996). <u>Trauma</u> (3rd ed.). Stamford, CT: Appleton & Lange.

Newberry, L. (Ed.). (1998). <u>Sheehy's emergency nursing: Principles and practice</u> (4th ed.). St. Louis: Mosby.

Rosen, P., & Barkin, R., Hayden, S. Shaider, J. & Wolfe, R. (1999). <u>The 5 minute emergency medicine consult</u>. Philadelphia: Lippincott Williams & Wilkins.

1. Which mechanism of injury should be transported immediately to the treatment area?
   a. Fall from a second story roof in an adult
   b. Stab wound to the left calf with no bleeding or pain
   c. Gunshot wound to the right hand 12 hours prior to arrival
   d. Crush injury of the distal phalanx of right second finger

2. Which patient in question 1 would be considered a level 1 in the ESI 5-Level triage system?

3. An intoxicated woman falls from a truck going 30 mph. The patient has abrasions and bruises over her face, arm, and legs. What is the most appropriate action for the triage nurse?
   a. Complete patient assessment in the triage area.
   b. Apply a soft cervical collar and complete patient assessment.
   c. Transport to the treatment area immediately.
   d. Clean the abrasions then transport to the treatment area.

4. Pediatric patients who are victims of pedestrian accidents are more likely to sustain significant injuries than adults because:
   a. Their size places their chest and abdomen closer to the bumper.
   b. They usually face the vehicle at the time of impact.
   c. They are smaller than adults are and more likely to be thrown.
   d. All the above.

5. A young male is found outside the triage area. He is unconscious and has blood on his chest and torso. His skin is pale, cool, and clammy. The most appropriate action for the triage nurse is:
   a. Get help to put the patient on a stretcher.
   b. Search the patient for identification.
   c. Call the police to locate the next of kin.
   d. Place paper bags on the patient's hands in case he was shot.

6. What level, based on the 5-level system, would the patient in question 5 be classified?
   a. 1
   b. 2
   c. 3
   d. 4
   e. 5

7. A 44 year old male patient is dropped on the ambulance ramp from a car that immediately drives off. Initial assessment reveals an unconscious patient with stridor. There is a gunshot wound noted on the left temple and chest. The first action for the triage nurse is:
   a. Open the airway
   b. Assess breath sounds
   c. Check the pulse
   d. Listen to heart sounds

8. Determine the appropriate priority for the following patients based on both the 3- and 5-level systmes.

Acuity	Patient
_______	33 year old male with amputation of the left index fingertip.
_______	89 year old female with obvious deformity of left upper arm. Vital signs are within normal limits.
_______	15 year old male involved in low speed motor vehicle collision. The patient is on a long spine board. Vital signs are within normal limits. There are no obvious injuries.
_______	75 year old male hit in head from a line drive during a high school baseball game. He does not remember what happened but complains of a severe headache.
_______	22 year old female with deformity of left foot after it is run over by a forklift. The patient complains of severe pain.

1. Review applicable trauma protocols for management of trauma in your facility.

2. Identify the location of equipment for spinal immobilization.

3. Discuss safety issues related to patients who have been 'dropped off' on the ambulance ramps or in nearby parking area. Review applicable policies and procedures for your facility.

Advanced Triage Exercises *chapter 37*

OBJECTIVES

After completing this chapter, you will be able to:

1. Prioritize patients with different complaints who present simultaneously to the triage area.

2. Prioritize multiple patients with similar complaints.

3. Assign a 5-level category for each example below.

Previous chapters discussed triage of a single patient with a specific complaint or problem. However, the triage nurse is often faced with triage of several patients simultaneously. Ability to sort these patients and determine which patient should receive care first depends on clinical assessment and analysis of information from a variety of sources. The decision may be based on the patient's appearance, chief complaint, focused assessment, or combination of these. This chapter presents a series of triage situations that allow you to determine priority of care when presented with more than one patient.

CHIEF COMPLAINT

Review the following groups of chief complaints. Determine which patient should be seen first based on chief complaint. This exercise allows you to select who should come to the front of the 'assessment line." Explain your rationale for each decision.

Group A
- 75 year old patient with sudden loss of vision
- 24 year old patient with obvious deformity left forearm.
- 34 year old patient with severe left flank pain

Priority Ranking and Rationale
First

Second

Third

Group B

- 16 year old male with sudden onset testicular pain

- 30 year old male with hematuria for two weeks

- 50 year old male who has not urinated for 12 hours

Priority Ranking and Rationale
First

Second

Third

Group C

- 44 year old patient who fell from a second story roof

- 27 year old patient with a stab wound to the left calf with no bleeding or pain

- 38 year old patient with a gunshot wound of the right hand 12 hours prior to arrival

Priority Ranking and Rationale
First

Second

Third

Group D

- 4 year old child fell off a swing, has swollen right arm

- 6 year old child with fever 102° F orally

- 10 year old male with burn to the chest and right arm

Priority Ranking and Rationale
First

Second

Third

Group E

- Semi-conscious male who supposedly took several sleeping pills

- Confused belligerent male brought in from a long-term care facility

- Confused male with a history of seizures

Priority Ranking and Rationale
First

Second

Third

FOCUSED ASSESSMENT

Group A

Review the following patient scenarios. Determine which patient should be seen, first, second, and third. This exercise allows you to prioritize care after you complete the focused assessment. Provide your rationale for each decision.

Patient 1

A 2 year old is brought to the ED by his parents who tell you he has been hot and 'fifteen minutes ago he had a fit. He moved back and forth, he was breathing funny, and had foam in his mouth.' The toddler is now awake, but lethargic; skin is hot and dry. Rectal temperature is 104° F. Other vital signs are within normal limits. Parents have given the patient no medications in the past two hours.

Patient 2

A 5 year old with a ventricular shunt is brought to the triage area. The mother states the child has been sleeping a lot today and is now difficult to wake up. The child had a headache and vomited yesterday. The child now has snoring respirations and a pulse rate of 65. Skin color is pale and diaphoretic. The child responds with non-purposeful movement to painful stimuli

Patient 3

An 18 year old comes to the ED with headache and nausea after being struck in the head with a softball. The patient is alert and oriented. Skin is warm, dry, and has normal color. Vital signs are within normal limits, pupils are equal, and grip strength is equal. The patient walks without any problems and answers questions in a clear, easy to understand voice. The patient has no significant medical history and takes no medications.

Priority Ranking and Rationale
First

Second

Third

FOCUSED ASSESSMENT

Group B

Review the following patient scenarios. Determine which patient should be seen, first, second, and third. Provide your rationale for each decision.

Patient 1

A 75 year old female complains of tearing pain between her shoulder blades and numbness in lower extremities. She is pale, diaphoretic, and has weak pulses in the lower extremities. She tells you she thinks she is going to die.

Patient 2

A 55 year old male presents with sharp, right-sided chest pain for two days. He has had a cold for the past week with fever, and productive cough. The patient has decreased breath sounds on the right base. His temperature is 101° F, pulse 120, blood pressure is 140/88, respiratory rate 28, pulse oximetry 94%. Skin is warm ,dry and has normal color.

Patient 3

A 26 y.o construction worker complains of severe lower back pain with numbness of the right leg for 48 hours. Sudden pain started after lifting a heavy object two days ago. Skin is warm and dry. Vital signs are within normal limits.

Priority Ranking and Rationale

First

Second

Third

Group C

Review the following patient scenarios. Determine which patient should be seen, first, second, and third. Provide your rationale for each decision.

Patient 1

A 14 year old female is brought to the ED after she fainted during cheerleading rehearsal. The outside temperature is 96° F. She alert with hot, dry skin. Her lips are dry and her skin is flushed. She complains of severe weakness. Vital signs are pulse 124, blood pressure 96/58, and temperature 100° F.

Patient 2

A 64 year old male complains of swollen feet for three days. Outside temperature is 94° F. He has worked 8 to 9 hours a day for the past three days in his garden. He is alert and oriented and denies any medical problems. His vital signs are within normal limits and his breath sounds are normal. Skin is warm and dry.

Patient 3

A 2 month old is brought to the ED by his aunt who has been babysitting while the mother is on vacation. She has kept the infant inside for the past four days due to the severe heat wave in the area. She says the baby is not taking his bottle well and is fussy and irritable. There is also a fine rash over the baby's trunk and back. The aunt does not have air conditioning and wonders if the baby is too hot. The child is lethargic with skin that is flushed, hot, and dry. Temperature is 102.6° F, pulse is 145, and the respiratory rate is 48.

Priority Ranking and Rationale
First

Second

Third

ADVANCED TRIAGE TEMPLATES

Use the following templates to create your own scenarios based on the standards in your institution.

Case A

Across-the-Room Assessment

____

____

____

Case B

Across-the-Room Assessment

____

____

____

Case C

Across-the-Room Assessment

____

____

____

Primary/Secondary Assessment

Use this template to develop scenarios for adult patients with illness as well as injuries.

Assessment	Case A	Case B	Case C
Airway			
Breathing			
Circulation			
Disability			
Expose			
Full Set of Vital Signs			
Five Interventions			
Facilitate Family Presence			
Give Comfort Measures			
History			
Head-to-Toe Assessment			
Inspect Posterior Surfaces			

ENA (2000) *Trauma Nursing Core Course* (Fifth Ed.). Des Plaines, IL: Author.

Pediatric Patients

CIAMPEDS

Use this template to create scenarios for multiple pediatric patients that challenge the learner to identify the patient with the most critical need.

Assessment	Case A	Case B	Case C
Complaint			
Immunizations			
Allergies			
Past medical History			
Events around illness			
Diet or diapers			
Symptoms associated with illness			

ENA (1999). *Emergency Nursing Pediatric Course* (Second Ed.). Des Plaines, IL: Author.

SAVE A CHILD

Use this template to create scenarios for multiple pediatric patients that challenge the learner to identify the patient with the most critical need.

Assessment	Case A	Case B	Case C
Skin			
Activity			
Ventilation			
Eye Contact			
Abuse			
Cry			
Heat			
Immune System			
Level of Consciousness			
Dehydration			

Aloha Chapter, Hawaii ENA.

Glossary

Across-the-room assessment – visual assessment of the patient's general well-being, airway, breathing, circulation, and disability. Acuity category may be assigned at this time.

Acuity – severity of illness or injury as well as the potential for complications related to the illness or injury.

Acuity category – category assigned to the patient to identify their acuity or need for medical attention.

AICD – automatic implanted cardioverter defibrillator

AMA – against medical advice. The patient refuses care or leaves the facility against the advice of the physician.

Aura – sensation of light, warmth, or sounds that precede a migraine headache or epileptic seizure.

AVPU – acronym used to classify the patient's level of consciousness; alert, responds to voice, responds to pain, or unresponsive.

Avulsion – soft tissue wound in which the wound edges cannot be approximated, tearing away of a portion of the soft tissue.

Battle's Sign – ecchymosis behind the ear over the mastoid process. May indicate basilar skull fracture of the posterior fossa.

CIAMPEDS – acronym for assessment of the pediatric patient – chief complaint, immunizations, allergies, medical history, events surrounding the illness, diet/diapers, and symptoms associated with the illness.

Costovertebral angle (CVA) – one of two angles that outlines a space over the kidney-at the intersection of the spinal column and the twelfth rib.

COBRA – Consolidated Omnibus Reconciliation Act. See EMTALA.

Crepitus – dry, crackling sound; bony crepitus is the sound heard when fractured bone ends rub together.

Dysphagia – difficulty swallowing

Dypsphonia – difficulty speaking, e.g. hoarseness

Ecchymosis – bluish areas of discoloration of skin or mucous membranes which are larger than petechiae

Eclampsia – when the patient with PIH or pre-eclampsia has a seizure, the condition is called eclampsia. Can be life-threatening. Delivery reverses the condition.

EMTALA – Emergency Medical Treatment and Active Labor Act. Federal legislation to prevent patient dumping.

Envenomation – injection of snake or insect venom into the body

Expected date of confinement (EDC) – an estimate of date for child's birth calculated by counting back three months from the date of the last menstrual period then adding seven days.

Extraocular Eye movements (EOMs) – movement of the globe in various directions; movements are under control of cranial nerves III, IV, and VI which innervate the six eye muscles.

Family – an individual's support system; may include, but is not limited to, relatives, friends, and significant others.

Flank – side of the body from the ribs to the ischium of the hip; similar in definition to loin which is the posterior area of the body from the chest to the pelvis.

Focal Seizure – seizure activity limited to one area of the body – arm, leg, face, eyes.

Gestation – time from fertilization of the egg to birth; gestational age refers to the age of the fetus in utero at any given time.

Grand Mal Seizure – generalized tonic-clonic motor seizure.

Hyphema – hemorrhage into the anterior chamber of the eye, usually caused by blunt injury.

Joint Commission on Accreditation of Healthcare Organizations (JCAHAO) – organization that develops standards for patient care in healthcare organizations.

Medical Screening Exam (MSE) – medical exam mandated by EMTALA to rule out an emergency medical condition. Must be done before there is any discussion of finances.

Mistriage – assignment of an acuity level that is higher or lower than necessary for a specific patient.

MIVT – acronym for mechanism of injury, injuries, vital signs, and treatment used by prehospital personnel to communication information to hospital personnel.

Neonate – birth to 4 weeks of age. If the infant is preterm, he/she remains a neonate until the expected due date plus 28 days.

Orthostatic Vital signs – blood pressure and pulse taken before and after change in position – lying to sitting, lying to standing, or sitting to standing.

Over-triage – assignment of an acuity level that is higher acuity than necessary

Paresthesia – burning, prickling, numbness, or other abnormal sensation.

Petechiae – small (less than 3 mm in diameter), reddish, purple, macular lesions. They are the result of hemorrhages within the dermal or submucosal layers.

Poikilothermy – the patient's temperature becomes the same as the environmental temperature.

Pregnancy Induced Hypertension (PIH) – also called pre-eclampsia. Characterized by hypertension, edema, and proteinuria. Condition is known as eclampsia if the patient has a seizure.

Primary Assessment – assessment of the airway, breathing, circulation and level of consciousness (disability) to identify conditions that are immediately life-threatening.

Protocol – guideline for assessment and/or treatment of patients with a specific condition, complaint, or problem. Usually approved for use in a specific institution or organization.

Pulsus Paradoxus – abnormal decrease in systolic blood pressure with inspiration. Associated with severe asthma, cardiac tamponade, and severe heart disease.

Purpura – ecchymotic areas reflecting blood in the skin or mucosal membranes. This may occur with several different bleeding disorders, meningococcemia, or sepsis.

Raccoon eye's – ecchymosis around the eyes. May indicate basilar skull fracture of the anterior fossa.

SANE – Sexual Assault Nurse Examiner; nurse who receives special training for assessment of the sexual assault victim.

Save-a-child – mnemonic developed by the Aloha Chapter (Hawaii ENA) for assessment of the pediatric patient – skin, activity, ventilation, eye contact, abuse, cry, heat, immune system, level of consciousness, and dehydration.

Secondary Assessment – patient assessment from head to toe to identify all injuries.

Subcutaneous emphysema – air beneath subcutaneous tissue in the interstitial spaces. Occurs most often in the chest and neck from an air leak secondary to disruption of the larynx, trachea, or bronchi.

Status Epilepticus – tonic-clonic seizure that continues without recovery or interruption. Usually lasts more than an hour.

Trauma – Greek word that means wound. Used interchangeably with injury.

Triage – process used to determine urgency of need for emergency care based on assessment findings. The word triage means to sort or choose.

Under-triage – assignment of an acuity level that is lower than appropriate.

Appendix A
Triage Assessment Competency Guidelines

The competent triage nurse demonstrates the ability to:

1. Complete across-the-room assessment in 30 seconds or less.
   * General appearance, airway, breathing, circulation, and disability

2. Complete triage assessment in 5 minutes or less.

3. Adjust across-the-room assessment and triage assessment to the patient's age.

4. Adjust triage assessment to the patient's level of understanding.

5. Elicit pertinent subjective data.
   * Chief complaint
   * History of current event or illness
   * Pertinent past medical, surgical, and perinatal history
   * Allergies
   * Current medications
   * Immunization status
   * Last normal menstrual period

6. Collect pertinent objective data specific to the patient's condition and complaint.
   * Vital signs
   * Demonstrate use of equipment with ability to troubleshoot problems
   * Determine validity of noninvasive equipment monitoring values
   * Pulse—peripheral and apical
   * Respiratory rate and effort
   * Blood pressure—auscultated and palpated
   * Temperature—oral, rectal, and tympanic
   * Orthostalic vital signs (pulse and blood pressure)
   * Capillary refill
   * Pulse oximetry
   * Weight
   * Breath sounds
   * Skin signs
   * Peripheral motor and sensory examination
   * Visual acuity
   * Pupil exam—size, shape, reaction to light, and accommodation
   * Extraocular movements
   * Treatment prior to arrival

7. Assess pain utilizing appropriate pain scales for severity measurement.

8. Assess cultural, religious, and spiritual needs.

9. Identify learning limitations.

10. Recognize actual or potential threats to life, vision, and limb.

11. Identify emergent, urgent, and nonurgent conditions based on knowledge of normal and abnormal anatomy and physiology.

12. Assign appropriate triage acuity based on patient assessment and department guidelines.

13. Perform nursing interventions based on patient condition and department policy.
    - Apply ice, splints, dressing, cervical collar
    - Determine glucose level

14. Initiate nursing protocols based on patient assessment and department policy.
    - Fever protocol
    - X-ray protocol
    - Lab protocol

Appendix B
Adult Learning

Variation in how we process information and utilize new knowledge affects how we teach and how we learn. One individual may balance a checkbook to the penny, whereas another may round entries to the next highest dollar. You may set your clock 20 minutes ahead, whereas your spouse may set it to the exact time. These differences occur regardless of the work setting or the individuals involved. One nurse may organize the work area in a precise, predetermined pattern, whereas another may work blissfully and effectively in chaos and disorder. Preceptors must recognize and embrace these variations through sensitive communication and implementation of various teaching strategies.

Adult Learning Principles

As a preceptor, you can have a profound effect on the learner's professional knowledge and performance. You are teaching an adult with a wealth of life experience who is also an independent thinker. Adult learners have diverse learning needs, backgrounds, preferences, and skills. However, adult learners also share many traits and characteristics (see Table II-1). Motivation for learning varies with the learner. Learning may be driven by enjoyment, desire for self-improvement, or specific job requirements. To effectively teach an adult and change learner behavior, you must appreciate these unique characteristics and understand basic tenets of adult learning. Adult learners are self-directed and life-centered in their approach to learning. These individuals learn primarily from experience and maintain their ability to learn throughout life. Adults need to know why they should learn something and they generally want to learn something useful.

Table II-1. Characteristics of Adult Learners
• Fear failure or inadequacy
• Respond better to positive reinforcement
• Enjoy success
• Prefer active participation
• Appreciate recognition of past experiences
• Dislike wasting time
• Enjoy a variety of teaching methods
• Participate in the learning process
• Have certain expectations of the learning environment

Thinking Patterns

Thinking patterns determine how we approach a problem. Abstract thinkers, concrete thinkers, sequential thinkers, and random thinkers approach teaching and learning in distinctly different ways (see Table II-2). Individuals usually exhibit strong preferences for one or two patterns; however, a mix of all patterns may be seen. As a preceptor, you should identify your own predominant thinking pattern as well as the pattern preferred by the learner. With this knowledge, you can tailor your teaching to the individual. For example, the individual who is a sequential thinker learns best with step-by-step teaching strategies.

Table 2. Abstract and Concrete Thinking Characteristics		
Pattern	**Characteristics**	**Assets/Liabilities**
Abstract Thinker	•Visualizes ideas and concepts •Conceives ideas •Uses intuition, intellect, and imagination—things are not always as they seem	•Is a creative problem solver but may come up with grandiose ideas that are not always practical •Can lose sight of the problem while imagining the solution
Concrete Thinker	•Uses sight, smell, touch, taste, and hearing. •Focuses on the here and now •Sees no hidden meaning—things are what they are	•Can miss subtle clues •Develops instinct slowly or not at all •Better at solving the obvious problems but is not good at coming up with ways to prevent problems from recurring
Sequential Thinker	•Uses linear thinking and a step-by-step approach •Prefers to plan •Likes to follow directions	•Gets down to the basics •Follows plans and procedures •Wants simple answers to complex questions and usually resists change
Random Thinker	•Organizes thoughts in chunks, usually skipping steps •Is impulsive and spontaneous •Has no plan, but usually gets things done	•Is a creative problem solver •Is good at initial program design •Does not follow through with details •Often alters plans or designs the plan to fit personal preference

Learning Styles

Recognized patterns of learning include brain dominance, multiple intelligence learning, and Kolb's theory of learning. An overview of each pattern is provided to help you adapt your preceptor techniques to different learners. As you review this material, consider your own preferences for learning. The pattern you prefer for learning strongly affects how you teach. Awareness of your personal preferences allows you to modify your instruction techniques to fit the learner while still utilizing your own inherent talents.

Brain dominance is based on the theory that individual thoughts and actions are determined predominantly by the actions of only one cerebral hemisphere.

- *Right brain dominance* is characterized by intuition and the use of patterns rather than focusing on details. Individuals who learn via right brain dominance see qualitative patterns clustered around images rather than viewing data organized sequentially. These individuals learn better when information is provided in patterns or chunks rather than step-by-step. For example, reviewing 39 individual steps of a procedure may cause this individual's attention to drift.

- *Left brain dominance* is characterized by use of logic to solve problems. Information is organized systematically. Skipping steps during procedural checks or providing impromptu quizzes may cause stress for this type of individual.

Multiple intelligence learning categorizes learning into seven distinct categories or processes. Individuals usually exhibit strong preferences for one or two categories.

- *Linguistic* learners use words. They love reading, writing, telling stories, and playing word games. Learning tools should include books, tapes, dialogue, and discussion.

- *Logical-mathematical* learners use reasoning. Calculations, puzzles, and questioning appeal to these learners. Drug calculations can be fun for these learners.

- *Spatial* learners prefer images and pictures. Doodling, drawing, and visualizing characterize spatial learners. Presenting floor plans for your ED may help spatial learners better understand the triage process and patient flow.

- *Bodily kinesthetic* learners use somatic sensations (e.g., running, jumping, gesturing). Role playing, using drama, and providing hands-on, and tactile learning experiences appeal to these learners.

- *Musical* learners utilize rhythms and melodies (e.g., whistling, tapping, humming). Mnemonics or rhymes appeal to these learners.

- *Interpersonal* learners like to bounce ideas off other people. Group games, mentoring, and apprenticeships interest these learners.

- *Intrapersonal* learners think deep inside themselves. Self-paced projects and time alone are important to these learners. Give them time to digest information and consider the problem at hand.

Myers-Briggs Type Indicator is one of the most reliable and popular learning style theories. Four sets of learning preferences—extraversion/introversion, sensing/intuition, thinking/feeling, and judging/perceptive—define learning styles. The individual learner usually exhibits a preference for one type within each set.

- *Extraversion/introversion:* Extraverts find energy in things and people, whereas introverts want to connect subject matter and develop a framework.

- *Sensing/intuition:* Sensing people are detail oriented, whereas intuition people trust hunches and look for the big picture.

- *Thinking/feeling:* Thinking individuals value fairness, and feeling individuals value harmony.

- *Judging/perceptive:* Judging people are decisive and self-regimented; perceptive people are adaptive and spontaneous.

Instruction Techniques

Effectively communicating knowledge, expectations, and criticism is only one aspect of the preceptor role. As a preceptor, you facilitate the learning process by creating an environment that promotes acquisition of new knowledge. Use a variety of teaching strategies to maximize the learning experience. Table II-3 highlights the amount of learning that is typically derived from various strategies. The benefit to a specific individual may vary significantly if he or she has a strong preference for a given learning style and/or thinking pattern; however, most individuals learn best when several strategies are used.

Table II-3. Learning Strategies	
Percent of Learning	**Strategy**
10%	Reading the material
20%	Listening to the information
30%	Observing a demonstration
50%	Listening to an explanation of the procedure and then observing a demonstration
70%	Listening to the information, observing a demonstration, and discussing the procedure
90%	Listening to the information, observing a demonstration, discussing the procedure, and then performing the procedure

Orientation Program

Meet with your learner to establish a relationship and identify any strong learning preferences. Explain the entire orientation program so the learner knows what to expect. Identify goals and objectives for the learning experience so that you are both working toward the same goal. Plan a program that fits the learner's needs, considers course content, and uses dominant learning styles of the preceptor and the learner. Flexibility during orientation is essential so you can modify your techniques to meet the learner's needs and face any crises that may arise. It is critical that you provide positive, objective feedback throughout the learning experience.

Summary

Preceptors and learners are individuals with unique thinking and learning patterns. Recognizing and appreciating these characteristics enables you to modify your instructional techniques to meet the needs of each learner. As you develop in the preceptor role, don't forget that learning should be fun. Enjoy the experience!

References

American Heart Association. (1997). <u>Instructor's manual: Advanced cardiac life support</u>. Dallas: Author.

American Heart Association. (1997). <u>Instructor's manual: Basic life support</u>. Dallas: Author.

American Heart Association. (1997). <u>Instructor's manual: Pediatric advanced life support</u>. Dallas: Author.

Banner, J.M., & Cannon, H.C. (1997). <u>The elements of teaching</u>. New Haven, CT: Yale University Press.

Gardner, H. (1993). <u>Frames of mind: The theory of multiple intelligences</u>. New York: Harper Collins.

Jordan, K. (Ed.). (2000). <u>Emergency nursing core curriculum</u> (5th ed.). Philadelphia: Saunders.

Kennedy, M.M. (1999). Generations: When boomers meet cuspers, busters, and netsters. <u>Point of View, 37</u>(3), 5-7.

Knowles, M.S. (1970). <u>The modern practice of adult education</u>. New York: Associated Press.

Kolb, D.A. (1986). <u>User's guide for the learning style inventory</u>. Boston: McBer and Company.

Langer, E.J. (1997). <u>The power of mindful learning</u>. Reading, MA: Addison-Wesley.

Morgan, R.R., Ponticell, J.A., & Gordon, E.E. (1998). <u>Enhancing learning in training and adult education</u>. Westport, CT: Greenwood Publishing Group.

Myers, I.B., & McCaulley, M. (1985). <u>Manual: A guide to the development and use of the Myers-Briggs Type Indicator</u>. Palo Alto, CA: Consulting Psychologist Press.

Newberry, L. (Ed.). (1998). <u>Sheehy's emergency nursing: Principles and practice</u> (4th ed.). St. Louis: Mosby.

Sims, R.R., & Sims, S.J. (1995). <u>The importance of learning styles</u>. Westport, CT: Greenwood Press.

Appendix C
Continuing Education Information

ACCREDITATION

ENA is an Approver of continuing education. ENA's standards meet the required criteria for most State Boards of Nursing. The Emergency Nurses Association is recognized as a Provider of continuing education in nursing in the states of Alabama (Provider #ABNP0026) and California (Provider #CEP2322).

CONTINUING EDUCATION CREDITS

The processing fee for this independent study is $50. To receive a certificate verifying your continuing education contact hours, complete the Chapter Checklist and the CECH Course Evaluation Form. Submit these documents, along with a check (payable to Emergency Nurses Association) in the amount of $50 to:

> Emergency Nurses Association
> Education Department
> 915 Lee Street
> Des Plaines, Illinois 60016-6569

Please complete the following information and mail this form, the Chapter Checklist and payment in the amount of $50, to the above address.

Name: ____
(as you want it to appear on your certificate)

Street Address:____

City:__________________ State:____________ Zip Code:__________

Rating Scale: Excellent = 4   Good = 3   Fair = 2   Poor = 1

Overall Evaluation:
1. How well did this program achieve its goals?__________
2. How well did the program meet your educational needs?__________
3. Rate the overall content.__________
4. Rate the quality of your Preceptor.__________
5. How would you rate the overall quality of the program?__________
6. If there are modules that did not meet your needs, please identify below:
   Comments:____

(This form may be duplicated.)

CHAPTER CHECKLIST

Chapter	Chapter Title	CECH Clinical	CECH Other	Preceptor Signature	Date Completed
1	Triage Overview		1.2		
2	Triage Assessment		3.0		
3	Documentation		1.2		
4	Legal Issues		1.2		
5	Customer Service		1.2		
6	Cultural and Religious Considerations		1.2		
7	Violence		2.0		
8	Disaster Triage		1.2		
	Total CECH Category Other		**12.2**		

Chapter	Chapter Title	CECH Clinical	CECH Other	Preceptor Signature	Date Completed
9	Universal Triage Parameters	1.2			
10	Abdomen / Pelvis	1.8			
11	Abuse and Neglect	2.0			
12	Back	1.2			
13	Bites and Stings	1.2			
14	Burns	1.2			
15	Chest	2.0			
16	Cold-Related Conditions	1.0			
17	Confusion	1.0			
18	Ear	1.0			
19	Extremity				
20	Eye				
21	Fever				
22	Head				
23	Heat-Related Conditi				
24	Mouth				
25	Neck				
26	Nose				
27	Obstetric Patients				
28	Psychiatric Complaints				
29	Respiratory Complaints				
30	Seizure				
31	Sexual Assault				
32	Skin Problems				
33	Surface Wounds	1.2			
34	Throat	1.0			
35	Toxicities	1.8			
36	Trauma	2.0			
37	Advanced Triage Exercises	2.0			
	Total Clinical CECH	**40.0**			
	Total CECH for Program	**52.2**			

Preceptor Name:_____________________________ Title:_____________________________

Facility Name:____ Date:_______________

(This form may be duplicated.)

Appendix D
Comprehensive Triage Standards

ANA Standard
None

Specialty Standard
The emergency nurse triages each patient and determines the priority of care based on physical, developmental, and psychosocial needs, as well as factors influencing access to health care and patient flow through the emergency care system.*

Rationale
Triage facilitates the flow of patients through the emergency care system to ensure timely evaluation of patient needs.

The ENA believes that safe, effective, and efficient triage can be performed only by a registered professional nurse who is educated in the principles of triage and who has a minimum of 6 months' experience in emergency nursing.

EMERGENCY NURSES ASSOCIATION MEASURE-MENT CRITERIA

1. **Assessment:** A rapid, systematic collection of data relevant to each patient's chief complaint, age, cognitive level, and social situation is conducted to obtain sufficient information to determine patient acuity and any immediate physical or psychosocial needs.

Competent Level

- Performs focused assessment of chief complaint on each patient entering the emergency care system, collecting subjective and objective data.
- Assesses patients in a timely manner according to established triage criteria.
- Documents the triage assessment, including appropriate subjective and objective data.

Excellent Level

- Serves as a role model and resource person in the assessment phase of triage.
- Participates in development, implementation, and/or revision of triage assessment systems, such as age-specific guidelines and complaint-specific protocols.
- Participates in development, implementation, and/or revision of tools for documenting the triage assessment.

2. **Diagnosis:** Information gathered in the assessment phase is analyzed to determine the severity of physical, psychosocial, and educational needs.

Competent Level

- Differentiates the severity of the patient's condition.
- Identifies nursing diagnoses and/or collaborative problems when possible.
- Documents clinical impressions.

Excellent Level

- Recognizes nursing diagnoses and/or collaborative problems using atypical or subtle defining characteristics.
- Acts as role model and resource person for triage confirmation, identification of collaborative problems, and/or validation of nursing diagnoses.

3. Outcome Identification: Individualized expected outcomes are identified for each patient.

Competent Level

- Formulates outcomes relative to nursing diagnoses and/or collaborative problems, available resources, the patient's abilities, and input from the patient and other health care providers.
- Identifies and documents measurable objective criteria.

Excellent Level

- Addresses atypical presentations to identify patients at high risk for adverse outcomes.
- Acts as a role model and resource person for confirmation and validation of outcome identification.

4. **Planning:** The urgency of physical, psychosocial, and educational needs is determined, and the course of action is formulated to attain expected outcomes.

Competent Level

- Differentiates the urgency of the patient's problems and prioritizes access to care based on the patient's acuity.
- Directs the patient to the appropriate treatment area, based on assessment, diagnoses, outcome identification, and acuity.
- Communicates pertinent information to other health care providers.
- Documents the acuity and the individual plan of care.
- Identifies interventions to attain expected outcomes.

Excellent Level

- Anticipates the patient's needs and interventions, based on identification of actual and high-risk health problems.
- Acts as a role model and resource person for the planning phase of triage.

5. **Implementation:** Interventions are implemented as identified in the plan of care.

Competent Level

- Initiates independent nursing measures.

- Initiates diagnostic procedures per established triage protocols.

- Initiates treatment per established protocols, for example, antipyretics.

- Documents all interventions.

  - Communicates pertinent information to the patient and significant others.

  - Mobilizes additional resources as needed.

Excellent Level

- Participates in development and implementation of independent nursing measures and collaborative protocols.

- Identifies implementation practices requiring modification or change.

- Acts as a role model and a resource person for independent and collaborative interventions.

6. **Evaluation:** The patient's response to intervention is evaluated.

Competent Level

- Reassesses the patient according to the acuity and established procedures.

- Evaluates and documents the effectiveness of all interventions, as appropriate.

- Modifies the plan of care, acuity, and the expected outcome based on new information or changes in assessment data.

Excellent Level

- Acts as a role model and resource person for the evaluation phase of the triage process.

- Identifies nursing or system deficiencies that may impede adequate evaluation of the patient.

7. Medical Screening Examinations: The emergency nurse offers medical screening examinations as defined by institutional policies and state and federal regulations.

Competent Level

- Promotes access to care through appropriate screening of patients in accordance with the Emergency Medical Treatment and Active Labor Act (EMTALA) and state regulations.

Excellent Level

- Participates in the development of policies related to screening examinations.

- Coordinates staff education related to medical screening examinations.

Appendix E
Sample Documentation Forms

Wellstar Emergency Services **Nursing Documentation** ☐ Cobb ☐ Douglas ☐ Kenn ☐ Paulding

Name | Non-English Speaking? ☐ Spanish Other _______ | **ROOM**
☐ Hearing Impaired ☐ Interpreter Requested

Chief Complaint | **Age** | **Time** | **Date** | **Pvt MD**

Potential Threat	**Assessment** ☐ NAD	**Skin**	**Pulse Ox**	I Red
☐ None apparent ☐ Life ☐ Vision ☐ Limb ☐ Infant/Child *NOT* Appropriate for age	☐ Resp distress ☐ Chest Pain ☐ Suicidal ☐ OD ☐ Altered LOC ☐ Violent ☐ Obvious fracture ☐ Hemorrhage ☐ Burn/Blisters ☐ Severe Pain	☐ WNL ☐ Pale ☐ Flushed ☐ Cyanotic ☐ Diaphoretic		II Yellow III Green IV Orange

Appearance	**Arrival**	**Disposition**	**Signature**
☐ Alert ☐ Uncooperative ☐ Cooperative ☐ Unresponsive	☐ Ambulatory ☐ WC ☐ Police ☐ Carried ☐ Stretcher ☐ Alone	☐ Exam ☐ Assess ☐ Registration ☐ WR ☐ FastTrack ☐ LBS signed	

Time | **Allergies** ☐ NKDA ☐ Tape ☐ Latex ☐ Food ☐ Environmental (pollen/bees) | Wt _______ ☐ Measured | **Tetanus** ☐ ≤5yrs ☐ > 5 yrs
Ht _______ Asthma > 6yrs | ☐ Peds Immunizations UTD (Info discussed if not current)

How/Where	Blood Pressure	Pulse	Irregular	Resp	Temp	Pulse Ox

LMP_______ ☐ Birth Control Pills
NA → ☐ Menopausal ☐ Hysterectomy ☐ Depo-Provera
Pregnant? Y N UNK FHT _______ Due Date _______
Visual Acuity ☐ Glasses ☐ Contacts ☐ Implants ☐ Blind
Left _____ Right _____ Both _____ Corrected _____

Safety Equip: ☐ No ☐ Seatbelt ☐ Airbag ☐ Child Safety Seat ☐ Helmet ☐ Goggles ☐ Pads ☐ Unknown
Treatment PTA: ☐ Denies ☐ See DHR ☐ Immobilized ☐ Medications

PPMH: ☐ Denies ☐ Diabetes ☐ Cardiac ☐ High Cholesterol ☐ TB ☐ HTN ☐ Asthma ☐ COPD ☐ Infect Dx ☐
Seizures ☐ Stroke ☐ GB Dx ☐ Ulcers ☐ Thyroid ☐ Cancer ☐ Depression ☐ Chronic Pain
Past Surgical History: ☐ CABG ☐ Cholecystectomy ☐ Appendectomy
Other:

CURRENT MEDS (OTC, Rx, Herbal): ☐ See Medication Sheet ☐ Partial listing ☐ Dose/Schedule Unknown

Cultural/Religious/Spiritual/Psychosocial/Learning Needs:
None identified
List:

Social History: ☐ ETOH _______ (Occ QD)
☐ Cigarettes/cigar/pipe _____ ppd ☐ Chewing tobacco ☐ Snuff
☐ Drugs

Mark only those systems that apply to complaint or presenting symptoms.

		Surface Problems	**Pain Assessment**

Neurologic	Y	N	Respiratory	Y	N	Cardiac	Y	N	Skin	Y	N	Surface Problems	Scale	Faces
Alert			Cough Prod			Chest pain			Warm/Dry			☐ Laceration ☐ Abrasion		
Oriented X 3			Retractions			Epigastric			Diaphoretic			☐ Bruises ☐ Amputation		
+ LOC			Able to speak			Substernal			Hot Cool Cold			☐ Deformity ☐ Rash	Circle ↓	Check ↓
Dizzy			Dyspnea			Sharp Pressure Dull			Pale Flushed			Where	10	
Headache			Shallow			Radiates to:			Cyanotic				9	😞
Slurred speech			Stridor			JVD			Jaundice			Size	8	
Facial Asymmetry			Snoring						CRT:				7	😞
MAE			Orthopnea			**EENT**			**GYN GU**				6	
Weakness			Breath Side/Front/Back			Hoarse			Itching			Appearance	5	😐
RA LA RL LL			Sounds R L A P			Sore Throat			VB pds/hr:				4	
Sensory changes			Clear			R/L/B in appropriate column ↓			Dischg V P			Pulses ☐ Present	3	🙂
Blurred vision			Crackles			Eyes Red			Frequency			☐ Decreased ☐ Absent	2	
Photophobia			Wheezes			Eyes Draining			Retention			ROM	1	🙂
Pupils PERL			Decreased			Ear Drainage			**Gastrointestinal**			☐ Normal ☐ Decreased		
Brisk-B ? PERL R L			Abnormal			Nasal Drainage			N V D			Sensory	0	😀
Sluggish-S Size			Absent			Nose bleed			Color			☐ Normal ☐ Absent		
Pinpoint-PP Rxn						FB: Eye Ear Nose			Bleeding			☐ Decreased ☐ Increased		
									Frequency					

Protocols ☐ Fever Adult ☐ Fever Pediatrics ☐ Sprain ☐ Tetanus ☐ UTI ☐ Chest Pain ☐ Respiratory Distress ☐ Eye Injury ☐ Amputation ☐ Fracture

Triage Actions ☐ Cervical collar ☐ Ice ☐ Elevate ☐ Pressure dressing ☐ Splint | **Blood Sugar** | **Time** | **Updated Acuity Rating**
Other: | | | ☐ I Red ☐ II Yellow ☐ III Green

To Room @	To x-ray @	Assessed by	Time Date (if different from above)